On
Addiction

On
Addiction

DARIN WEINBERG

Insights
from
History,
Ethnography,
and Critical
Theory

Duke University Press
Durham and London 2024

© 2024 Duke University Press
All rights reserved
Project Editor: Livia Tenzer
Designed by Aimee Harrison and Courtney Leigh Richardson
Typeset in Warnock Pro by Copperline Book Service

Library of Congress Cataloging-in-Publication Data
Names: Weinberg, Darin, author.
Title: On addiction : insights from history, ethnography,
and critical theory / Darin Weinberg.
Description: Durham : Duke University Press, 2024. | Includes
bibliographical references and index.
Identifiers: LCCN 2024003244 (print)
LCCN 2024003245 (ebook)
ISBN 9781478030829 (paperback)
ISBN 9781478026587 (hardcover)
ISBN 9781478059813 (ebook)
Subjects: LCSH: Drug addiction—Social aspects. | Substance
abuse—Social aspects. | Drug addiction —Psychological
aspects. | Substance abuse—Psychological aspects. |
Drug addiction—Moral and ethical aspects. | Substance abuse
—Moral and ethical aspects. | Addicts—Social conditions. |
BISAC: SOCIAL SCIENCE / Sociology / General |
PHILOSOPHY / Movements / Critical Theory
Classification: LCC RC564 .O523 2024 (print) |
LCC RC564 (ebook) | DDC 362.29—dc23/eng/20240509
LC record available at https://lccn.loc.gov/2024003244
LC ebook record available at https://lccn.loc.gov/2024003245

Cover art: Egon Schiele, *Self-Portrait with Eyelid Pulled Down*,
1910. Chalk, brush, watercolor, and body color on brown
packing paper, 44.3 × 30.5 cm. Albertina, Vienna.

The chapters that follow are based on a selection of essays I've written over the past twenty-five years or so. They share their earliest origins in my PhD research at UCLA in the 1990s, which was conducted primarily under the guidance of Mel Pollner, Bob Emerson, and Harold Garfinkel and culminated in the book *Of Others Inside: Insanity, Addiction, and Belonging in America*. That said, though, and as might be imagined, my thinking has continued to evolve during this time. More importantly, the chapters that follow have all been written not simply as mere extensions or elaborations of themes I developed in that book but in direct response to a range of different debates that have been influential in addiction studies since that time, in the social sciences and beyond.

To the extent they have been crafted in the first instance as constructive contributions to a range of different debates, they are better understood as distinctly local products of these debates themselves rather than as derivatives of a fixed epistemic orthodoxy, theoretical outlook, or method of investigation. However, as I seek to make clear in the introduction, this does not mean they aren't supplementary to one another, mutually implicative, and mutually reinforcing. They certainly are. But as I also seek to make clear in the introduction, this should not be understood to reflect an orthodox commitment to one scientific paradigm or another but as a historically and culturally specific social achievement, an achievement forged under, and with respect to, particular institutional and intellectual conditions outside of which this achievement has very little meaning.

Indeed, the primary objective of this volume is to make the case that addiction science has been widely hobbled by fixed axiomatic commitments predicated on one or another established scientific paradigm, methodology, epistemology, or rationality. More specifically, I argue it is precisely a widespread commitment to their respective axiomatic orthodoxies that has often caused both social and medical scientists to find understanding addiction as a loss of self-control so elusive. Despite a robust cross-disciplinary consensus that the loss of self-control is the defining criterion of addiction, neither the social nor the medical sciences have made much headway in adequately providing for what in the world this really means to people.

Because they tend to see people as intrinsically self-interested cost-benefit analysts, social scientists have struggled to avoid also theorizing addiction and recovery from addiction as products of voluntary cost-benefit calculations. But if addiction is voluntary and rational, why not manage it with ordinary rewards and punishments, incentives and disincentives, rather than some kind of therapy? Conversely, because they tend to see human life as biomechanical, medical scientists have struggled to avoid theorizing addiction and recovery from addiction in biologically reductionist terms that provide rather poorly for the lived experiences of self-control, its loss, or its recovery among addicts themselves. The following chapters are devoted in different ways to clarifying what it actually means for addicts to exercise self-control, to lose it, or to once again recover it, and especially what these mean to addicts themselves.

More broadly, the chapters collected here reflect my efforts to expand the scope of how we think about addiction beyond generalizations regarding its neurological, psychological, or sociological substrates and into a more specific and particularist appreciation of the understandings that can be gleaned from historical, ethnographic, and critical theoretical forms of investigation. This is decidedly not an effort to displace orthodox orientations to addiction science but rather to supplement them and to contextualize them. As a sociologist, I have long believed that much novel insight can come not only from attending to the historical and ethnographic realities that yield addictions themselves but also by attending, reflexively, to the historical and ethnographic realities that have shaped our own work as addiction scientists as such and in all our myriad guises.

This exercise has important consequences not only for addiction scientists but also for addiction counselors, politicians, policymakers, friends and families of addicts, addicts themselves, indeed everyone who would hope to foster therapeutic interventions over criminal prosecution and prohibition. If we are to genuinely help and empower people to overcome their addictions, we must understand in detail what addiction and recovery mean to them and why. And if we are to foster therapeutic over punitive interventions at the level of culture, law, and policy, we must be resourced with arguments that persuasively specify in detail what we are talking about and why. This has not yet been as effectively accomplished as I believe the following chapters allow. Moreover, I have come to believe that the limitations of received addiction science in this respect have deep roots in the histories of the disciplines devoted to the study of addiction. Therefore, our efforts must attend to these roots and we must be prepared to radically revise many of our most cherished assumptions concerning the sciences of addiction. And, more specifically, we must be prepared to radically revise many of our most cherished assumptions concerning things like the nature of our bodies, ourselves, our environments, and the diverse relationships we understand to connect these things to one another. It is precisely such revisions the reader will find in this book.

ACKNOWLEDGMENTS

Over the course of writing the chapters that comprise this book I have been influenced in many different ways by a broad collection of friends and colleagues, many of whom write specifically about addiction and many of whom do not. In alphabetical order, I would like to gratefully acknowledge the intellectual debt I owe to Pertti Alasuutari, Tammy Anderson, Doug Anglin, Patrick Baert, Howard Becker, Joel Best, David Bogen, David Bolton, Philippe Bourgois, Craig Calhoun, Nancy Chodorow, Peter Conrad, Fay Dennis, Cameron Duff, Griffith Edwards, Bob Emerson, Gil Eyal, Kathryn Fox, Suzanne Fraser, Harold Garfinkel, Erich Goode, Emile Gomart, Teresa Gowan, Robert Granfeld, Monica Greco, Jay Gubrium, Nick Heather, Matilda Hellman, John Heritage, Jim Holstein, Peter Ibarra, Bruce Johnson, Annemarie Jutel, Helen Keane, Larry King, John Kitsuse, James Laidlaw, Mike Lynch, Doug Maynard, Gale Miller, David Moore, Sheigla Murphy, James Nicholls, Andrew Pickering, Mel Pollner, Geoff Raymond, Craig Reinarman, Gerda Reith, Robin Room, Marsha Rosenbaum, David Rudy, Joe Schneider, Bryan Turner, Nicole Vittelone, Scott Vrecko, Ivan Weinberg, and Phil Withington.

It has been an absolute pleasure to work with Elizabeth Ault and Benjamin Kossak at Duke University Press throughout the review process. I would also like to thank Livia Tenzer, my project editor at the press, for her oversight of the production process. The book is now a much more lucid and readable text thanks to her efforts. Thanks also to Aimee Harrison for her inspired artistic design of the book and to Courtney Leigh Richardson for shepherding it to the finish line.

The philosopher Ludwig Wittgenstein once suggested that his writing style often involved coming at a collection of problems from different analytic angles and thereby revealing their multiple theoretical facets as well as their multifaceted relationships with each other. Something like this logic is behind my own argument for the value of bringing these writings together into a single volume. They exhibit more than twenty-five years of my reflections on various aspects of the social nature and social explanation of addiction and the history of others' important considerations of these questions. However, taken together they also exhibit the intellectual gestalt that unites them much more effectively than any of them considered on their own could possibly be hoped to. The fact that these essays are supplementary to one another, mutually implicative and mutually reinforcing in a variety of ways, grounds my argument that the whole of this collection is greater than the sum of its parts.

More specifically, Isaiah Berlin famously distinguished between foxes and hedgehogs in his only slightly whimsical account of the intellectual styles of major thinkers in the Western philosophical canon. I hope readers will agree that these essays convey something of my aspiration and, more substantively, the specific collection of techniques I have adopted, to endeavor to forge a distinctive union between these two styles of thought. For those unfamiliar with Berlin's distinction, it is essentially a contrast between scholars, foxes, who seek to provide reflections on a variety of specific themes, and hedgehogs, or those who seek to tackle one particular major theme. On the one hand, these essays cover a fairly broad collection of topics: the sociological canon; key sociocultural contexts within which major chapters in addiction science took shape; addiction, experience, and the body; the interface between medical and social understandings of addiction; posthumanism and addiction; and others. On the other hand, these essays all reflect an enduring meditation on the question of how we might more adequately provide conceptually for addicts' putative alienation from their actions and experiences or their loss of self-control to addictions and the ethical ramifications thereof.

This chapter provides a holistic account of the argument that links the following chapters into a coherent, if multifaceted, intellectual position concerning the social nature and social explanation of addiction. The argument is fundamentally focused on briefly describing how later chapters serve to dissolve various antinomies that have long limited research not only in the social sciences of addiction but throughout the addiction sciences more generally. As will be seen, these antinomies include those that oppose free will to determinism, mind to body, ethics to science, rationality to emotion, culture to nature, particular to universal, practice to theory, subjectivism to objectivism, micro to macro levels of analysis, and presentist and historicist orientations to analysis.

In addition to dissolving antinomies that have long fettered research on addiction, the book is devoted to the allied project of forging syntheses, most centrally among history, ethnography, and critical theory but also between the clinical and the social sciences. This chapter demonstrates how addiction provides an ideal empirical vehicle for the articulation of these syntheses. To the extent it is understood to entail a loss of self-control over one's behavior, addiction requires an intellectual framework supple enough to provide for movements into and out of self-control, the various social and natural processes that may influence these movements, the historical contexts within which these topics have variously become matters of widespread concern, and the ethical ramifications that follow from taking these matters seriously. At its core, the framework I defend combines an ethnomethodologically informed, posthumanist orientation to the history and sociology of science and clinical care with recent insights drawn from the anthropology of ethics. However, it also integrates insights from a variety of other relevant lines of inquiry, including analytic philosophy and the sociology of emotions. In addition to facilitating achievement of the intellectual objectives outlined here, these orientations to research highlight the variable exigencies that confront and constrain self-governance, science, and clinical work in particular cases without thereby reducing these to mere effects of those exigencies.

As many of the following chapters note, mainstream addiction science is today largely polarized between, on the one hand, those who argue that addiction is a brain disease biomechanically caused by pathological neuro-adaptations to prolonged exposure to addictive drugs or activities and, on the other hand, those who argue that addiction is a form of voluntary activity freely engaged by those who are called addicts (see Heather et al. 2022).

Brain disease scientists highlight the clinical facts that addictions cause immense suffering and often defy the efforts of addicts themselves, their significant others, and clinicians to make sense of them as freely engaged activities. They further note the results of laboratory research that show in some considerable detail the kinds of structural and functional changes that brains undergo as a result of exposure to drugs and other addictive substances or practices. Finally, they insist that it is unethical to punish people for behavior they cannot control and that the only ethical remedy for addiction is the provision of clinical care.

Those who argue that addicts do not exhibit a loss of self-control point to the facts that addiction appears to be incentive sensitive, or at least to some extent consistent with cost-benefit calculations. They insist that the language of disease stigmatizes and disempowers people with drug problems, suggesting they are incapable of overcoming their problems without professional medical intervention. And they point to the ubiquity of controlled drug use, the fact that many addicts "mature out" of their addictions without clinical intervention and that drug problems appear to be fundamentally linked to the social contexts in which people live. While they consistently oppose blaming addicts for their problems, choice theorists are less clear about how exactly this is to be avoided if addiction is a free choice (see Berridge 2022).

This antinomy between free will and determinism in addiction science stems from the fact that both disease and choice theorists seek to provide generic models of addiction. This prevents them from theorizing the labile movements into and out of self-control that are the hallmark of addiction and recovery in practice. Disease theorists, for their part, are often axiomatically blocked from taking freedom seriously by their biomechanically reductionist orientation to explanation. Conversely, choice theorists often struggle to articulate a persuasive justification for suspending default tendencies to hold ourselves and one another ethically accountable for our actions. This is because they are too often committed to the idea that all behavior not caused by brute physical force is necessarily free. The "addiction as akrasia" thesis comes closest to addressing these limitations in mainstream addiction science but because it too is cast in general terms, it cannot adequately provide for contingent movements into and out of self-control in actual cases.

I argue that by drawing upon theoretical resources provided by Michel Foucault, Harry Frankfurt, and Donald Davidson, these problems can be effectively overcome. Without fully rehearsing it in detail here, this argument shows how Foucault's thought on what he called "practices of freedom" furnishes some basic theoretical resources with which to capture the particularity of personal freedom and recovery from addiction in practice. Conversely, I show how Foucault's thought also provides for an exterior to ethical subjectivity that may occasionally intrude upon our lives in practice, thereby rendering our actions comparatively insulated from ethical accountability. I also show how Foucault's thought can be usefully refined in this regard by recourse to Frankfurt's ruminations on the practicalities of free will (or distinguishing in practice those mental contents "internal" to the self and self-control from those that are "external," harmful or threatening to particular selves). The argument is further refined with recourse to Davidson's famous reflections on mental compartmentalization, the principle of charity, and the difference between reasoned/willed action and behavior that is causally determined by mental structures but is nonetheless unreasoned/unwilled. In sum, the argument demonstrates that in practice freedom, addiction, and recovery from addiction are best understood in terms of the details of particular people's lives rather than generically through the generalizations found in most mainstream addiction science.

Mind and Body

The intellectual context in which the first major sociological contribution to the study of addiction was formulated heavily encouraged adoption of a rather rigid dichotomy between bodily and mental perception. In his classic sociological theory of addiction, Alfred Lindesmith argued that human perception is divided into the body's brute response to physical stimuli and the mind's active, conscious, and symbolic interpretation of that stimuli. Hence, for addiction to arise, addicts must reflectively interpret their physiological withdrawal symptoms specifically as withdrawal symptoms and self-consciously use heroin to alleviate those symptoms. Much like the choice theories mentioned previously, this argument makes it difficult to understand how a learned pattern of perception and behavior could ever be experienced as beyond the addict's control—that is, suffered rather than chosen. And also like other choice theories, Lindesmith's approach makes it difficult to understand why addiction should warrant suspension of our default tendencies to hold ourselves and one another ethically accountable for our actions.

In part to overcome these challenges, I have adapted Pierre Bourdieu's concept of habitus. This concept refers to embodied practical and perceptual dispositions that are acquired through practical engagement with particular social environments and facilitate competent participation in those environments. My argument has been that when some of these dispositions come to seriously conflict with dispositions with which actors are more inclined to self-identify, they come to be experienced in Frankfurt's terms as "external" to the self and as afflictions thereof. This approach has the consequence of shifting theoretical attention away from linguistic dispositions to symbolically interpret brute physical stimuli, and the mind-body dualism thereby assumed, and toward the specific practical environments in and for which people come to learn to use drugs or engage in prospectively addictive activities in practice. What once might have been widely known as reflective mental activities are here understood as largely prereflective, prediscursive, embodied, environmentally shaped and situated habits. The body ceases to be understood as an objective biomechanical system about which we might subjectively learn and is specified instead, in line with Bourdieu's and Bruno Latour's (2004) groundbreaking approaches, as a linked set of mutable media through which we subjectively learn and subjectively develop.

In a particularly incisive study of the "odor kits" that perfume makers use to train "noses" to detect progressively subtler aromatic contrasts, Latour (2004) makes a strong empirical case for what I call psychosomatic subjectivity. Latour goes a considerable distance toward creating a conceptual space within which addiction might be construed as an acquired but nonetheless fully embodied form of subjectivity. By retaining a focus on the subjective or lived sentient body, Bourdieu and Latour accommodate much of what choice theorists seek to achieve by narrowing the distance between addiction and normal learning processes. But although they write of the multiplicity of environments within which bodies subjectively learn to be affected, they do not explicitly address the multiplicity of the body itself—as not just an articulated medium for learning to be affected but a linked set of media for doing so. This limits their sensitivity to the potentials for embodied conflicts and/or afflictions like addiction.

Ethics and Science

The tendency of mainstream addiction science to seek ethically neutral generalizations regarding addiction and recovery systematically distances it from the details of particular people's lives. While mainstream addiction science is generally cast as ethically detached and universal, therapeutic work with addicts instead tends to require particularistic orientations to the aspirations, attitudes, challenges, opportunities, and aptitudes of specific addicts and an ethical engagement with them as collaborators in recovery as opposed to scientific or ethical detachment. All my work has been attentive to the need to allow scientific space for the specificity of particular people, their communities, and their histories as well as being emphatically critical of the notion that science can, even in principle, be ethically disengaged.

On the historical front, I have been more concerned to write genealogies of particular fragments of the present than general narratives concerning the present or the past. This has involved comparative attention to similarities and differences among diverse times and places more than efforts to unearth their shared essences. Similarly, on the ethnographic front, I have sought to highlight similarities and differences among diverse communities and, indeed, the diversity of those who belong to these communities more than generalizations regarding them. Some may wish to argue that the only alternative to scientific generalizations are unrepresentative and ad hoc anecdotes and that the only alternative to ethical detachment is bias. I do not share this wish, and I believe the attention given to diversity, contingency, and particularity among proponents of the comparative case-study approach to historical and ethnographic empirical research is every bit as scientific as research cast in terms of general laws and/or causal mechanisms (see Calhoun 1998; Kandil 2022). I also argue that ethical engagement is, in practice, an inevitable feature of all scientific research and is not necessarily equal to bias.

As I have said, the framework I defend combines an ethnomethodologically informed, posthumanist orientation to the history and sociology of science and clinical care with recent insights drawn from the anthropology of ethics. Whereas received research usually casts rules only as devices for regulating social action, ethnomethodology has long highlighted how, by the active observance and invocation of rules, social action is rendered at all intelligible as reasoned action, let alone conventional or unconventional (see Garfinkel 1967; Heritage 1984; Maynard and Heritage 2022). Moreover, ethical accountability is not occasioned only intermittently when specifically ethical rules are violated but is an indispensable feature of the coordination of social interaction wherever it is found. Some strands of posthumanist scholarship provide usefully detailed understandings of the real-time constitution of both reasoned human and unreasoned nonhuman agency in practice and hence a nuanced scientific orientation to how in practice we might account for movements into and out of self-control and, in turn, movements into and out of ethical accountability (see Weinberg 2005). This kind of research highlights how the symptoms of addictions and indeed the disorders those symptoms indicate are variously constituted not in people's minds or brains considered in social isolation but in the details of ongoing social interaction.

More specifically, it shows that people's rights and/or obligations to such things as work, hospitalization, social services, trust, or the forbearance of their associates are in practice established not once and for all and with respect to fixed legal, medical, psychiatric, or social identities but provisionally through the situated evaluations and reevaluations of their myriad accountabilities, abilities, and disabilities across the range of settings within which they participate. I believe this is a crucially important scientific insight with far-reaching ramifications for addiction policy. If we are to claim that people diagnosed with addictions are entitled to special assistance, it is indispensable that we be able to both warrant that special assistance and empirically demonstrate the nature of their special needs. The proposed scientific framework transcends the contextually indiscriminate models of disorder provided by medicine and the "psy-" professions to demonstrate the social interactional constitution of disability across diverse settings. It thereby provides a more empirically nuanced linkage of specific addictions and the myriad types of social assistance they might be held to warrant. Though focused in the first instance on the detailed scientific analysis of people's practices, this type of research also promises insights of considerable value to those seeking to empirically ground addiction treatment, policy, and ethical reform agendas.

Rationality and Emotion

My earliest forays into considering the relationship between rationality and emotion were focused on symbolic interactionist accounts of addiction. In many of the following chapters, I develop a critique of the mind-body dualistic accounts of meaningful emotions, like desire or craving, often proffered by symbolic interactionists. This critique is based on the argument that these accounts effectively eviscerate emotion by construing its meaning as wholly cognitive and disembodied. As I show, by requiring that the meaning of emotion be uniformly cast in terms of reflective, symbolic, and rational interpretations of brute physiological experiences, these accounts fail to provide for meaningful emotions that have not been consciously interpreted or rationally evaluated and, hence, that might sometimes be seen to challenge our rational reflections. As an alternative, I conceptualize emotions as embodied, prereflective, and prediscursive dispositions to perceive and/or act in particular kinds of ways that we have learned through participation in various practical contexts. Whether or not we self-identify with our emotions, or indeed any of our habituated orientations to experience and activity, is not a fait accompli. Instead, as the philosopher Harry Frankfurt has argued, it is a matter of second order or meta-evaluation.

Symbolic interactionist accounts that speak to the role of emotions in addiction emphasize the mental interpretation of physiological experiences to an extent that sometimes obscures how the meaning of addictions is shaped in the first instance not by symbolic interpretations but by the ways we have learned to use drugs and other putative objects of addiction in particular practical contexts. However, the symbolic interactionist studies that speak to the role of rationality in addiction, much like those in anthropology, tend to be rather modest in their claims—casting rationality largely in terms of culturally relative cost-benefit analyses. This might also be said of many of the choice theorists of addiction. Most have now abandoned the idea that addictions are no more than rational choices based on stable preferences. In place of orthodox rational choice theory, many have followed theorists such as George Ainslie (1992) in arguing that addicts hyperbolically discount future costs and benefits—that is, the greater the expected immediacy and potency of a reward, the more one becomes prone to forsake their longer-term plans and preferences.

However, there is a community of addiction researchers who have embraced a much more philosophically robust orientation to rationality as composed of "all things considered" judgments based on explicit, universal, acontextual, and rule-based criteria. As is discussed in depth in chapter 5, these researchers posit a dual systems approach to decision-making wherein the first system is one that is variously characterized as fast, automatic, habituated, directly responsive to external cues, impulsive, affective, unintentional, unconscious, and energy efficient; and the second is slower, deliberative, conscious, self-directed, rational, intentional, rule-based, decontextualized, and energy inefficient. These systems are often referred to as system 1 and system 2, and I follow this convention. According to this approach, the locus of self-control is uniformly specified in terms of the more or less rationally coherent, holistic, and deliberative decision-making system 2. These arguments, however, often do not provide sufficiently for the manner in which type 2 decision-making processes are without exception based on foundations provided by type 1 processes. Not only are we sometimes prone to fetishize or repress our beliefs on the kinds of psycho-emotional grounds studied by psychoanalysts, but we may also distrust or dismiss the machinations of propositional rationality on other grounds as well. Indeed, as Wittgenstein (1953) taught us, conscious, rule-based deliberations are themselves always grounded in prediscursive dispositional competences forged in what he called particular forms of life—that is, ecologically bounded fields of activity.

Culture and Nature

Closely related to the antinomy between mind and body is the antinomy between culture and nature. With specific respect to addiction science, the concept of natural reward as relevant to biological survival and reproduction has been fundamental to neurological research on addiction. Conversely, the concept of culture has been fundamental to social research on addiction. Due primarily to interdisciplinary and intradisciplinary struggles for prestige and influence in the universities of the early twentieth century, starkly binary ontological oppositions between culture and nature have been installed as foundational conceptual commitments throughout both the social and natural sciences (Weinberg 2014).

The best-known source of this antinomy in the annals of social science methodology is the so-called *Methodenstreit*, or dispute over method, which embroiled some of Germany's finest social thinkers in a debate regarding the particular nature of social life and its amenability to the methods of the natural sciences. Thinkers such as Wilhelm Dilthey and Max Weber became figureheads for an intellectual movement that sought to decisively distinguish the social from the natural sciences on the grounds that their subject matters were irreducibly unique. Scholars argued that whereas the natural sciences study the inanimate universe and "lower life forms," social scientists study people. Unlike the behavior of the inanimate universe or lower life forms, human behavior is here said to be caused not by uniform laws but by sentient, creative subjects imbued with a cultural understanding of the worlds in which they live. Hence, the effort to grasp the nature of social life must begin with an appreciation of one's research subjects' own cultural understandings of their lives and circumstances.

Though over the years some social scientists have turned to Freudian and other psychodynamic theories, the more general trend has been opposed to presumptions of innate psychic processes (Chodorow 1999). Similarly, many social scientists in the first half of the twentieth century grew disenchanted with behavioral psychologists' refusal to acknowledge the role of meaning and creativity in human action and experience (Camic 1986). As physically and psychologically deterministic understandings of human action and experience were repudiated, social scientists increasingly viewed their subject matter as a domain unto itself, fundamentally irreducible to forces that were not themselves also cultural (Blumer 1969; Geertz 1973). These processes had immediate bearing on Lindesmith's formulation of addiction. They have also had fundamental influences on the work of symbolic interactionist, cultural anthropological, social psychological, economic, and philosophical research on addiction and drug use.

To be sure, the isolation of debates regarding the cultural dimensions of human life from those regarding our physical and psychic inheritances was never total. And, indeed, this isolation was always less pervasive in anthropology, where the collegial commingling of social and natural scientists was widely institutionalized through their sharing of a single academic department. But even when their research efforts are collaborative, cultural and physical anthropologists have always stood in uneasy analytic relation to one another. Though both strive to illuminate the causes and characteristics of the human condition, their theories and methods have often seemed to defy rigorous comparison with one another. Hence, the more popularly traveled debates on both sides of this antinomy have been those that do not seek to disturb the culture/nature divide (Latour 1993).

If ethnographers, historians, and other humanists have spoken to the natural dimensions of the human condition, they have overwhelmingly focused on the symbolic meaning and cultural function of natural objects rather than the details of their characteristic causal effects on human action and experience. As is argued in many of the following chapters, this has often imposed on social scientists a crippling antinomy between biomechanically deterministic understandings of addiction that cannot provide for the subjective discretion and, indeed, the genuine freedom of nonproblematic drug users or recovering addicts, on the one hand, and, on the other hand, an axiomatic humanist subjectivism in the social sciences of addiction that cannot escape an invariant commitment to the view that human action and experience are always, by definition, culturally meaningful and self-governed. Neither of these approaches can provide for what I have called an intellectual framework supple enough to capture movements into and out of self-control. I have sought to overcome the limitations of this axiomatic antinomy by recourse to the tradition of posthumanist social thought.

As we have seen, humanists tend to insist that the irreducible atoms of social life are inevitably human subjects—integrated, deliberative agents possessing interests and cultures that endow their worlds with meaning, value, and distinctive rationalities. Posthumanists worry that this imagery reifies human nature and denies the possibility of progressively reformulating or even modifying what it is to be human (Haraway 1991; Hayles 1999). Contrary to humanists, posthumanists do not treat human nature as intrinsically immutable but as something dynamically and diversely constituted through different configurations of practice within which actors, human or otherwise, mutually shape one another (Knorr-Cetina 1997; Latour 2005; Pickering 1995). Finally, eschewing reification, posthumanists historically and ethnographically examine situated practical action directly for clues as to how things are realized (literally made real) in any actual case.

Particular and Universal

Many scientists have long aspired to produce findings that are universal. More specifically, addiction science has routinely sought to argue on behalf of universally valid concepts of such things as rationality, the self, self-control, self-interest, choice, natural reward, neuroadaptations, and many others. My own work has been predicated on the belief that this approach is not so much flawed as incomplete in a variety of important respects. More specifically, because universals, by definition, do not change through history and thus appear immune to historical explanation, they tend to invite a disregard for history not only as an important source of influences on the phenomena we seek to understand but also as an important source of influence over the theoretical resources we adopt and with which we ourselves seek to construct our understandings. In short, they foster a blindness to the facts that both human behavior (including addiction and recovery) and our efforts to understand and/or explain human behavior are invariably embedded in and responsive to historical trends.

I should be clear that my effort has by no means been to critique the scientific aspiration to universality as such but to offer a reminder that even theories that proffer claims to universality are themselves perspectival—that is, they come from particular positions in history, including the history of the scientific disciplines within which their purveyors have been trained and to which they seek to contribute. Conversely, though, not even the most particular of events can be explained exclusively in terms of their particularity. To the extent we wish to understand how these events came about, we must situate them in more general, perhaps even sometimes universal, causal contexts.

Indeed, I have always argued that the generalizing sciences have certainly made important contributions to our understanding of addiction and recovery. However, it must not be forgotten that the loss and recovery of self-control take profoundly diverse forms. Both addiction and recovery are deeply personal matters that behoove close consideration of the particular aptitudes, opportunities, aspirations, and desires of particular people. To only briefly touch on some of the anomalies introduced by an overemphasis of universalizing in addiction science, we can begin by noting the now indisputable scientific fact that not everyone responds in the same way to drugs and other putative objects of addiction. Universalistic references to the intrinsically rewarding experiences of ingesting certain chemical compounds have been shown to be hopelessly callous to the diversity of effects drugs actually have not only on different people but also on the same people under different circumstances. Further, as is argued in several chapters, generic specifications of such matters as the reward circuitry of the human brain, differences between natural and unnatural rewards, and the nature of self-control, among others, have all been shown inadequate to the task of empirically understanding addiction and recovery in practice.

Theory and Practice

Like most science, addiction science is often devoted to transcending lay biases in the name of a more rigorous and epistemically legitimate understanding of the phenomena it considers. To note only one very prominent example, this can be seen in the almost complete consensus among addiction scientists that we must transcend the empirically erroneous lay bias that addicts are simply immoral and deserving of punishment rather than care. Though meritorious, this aspiration has too often been undergirded by a presumption that science is capable of completely transcending history and arriving to a space of purely theoretical reflection that is influenced only by ahistorical and universal standards of logic, evidence, and/or scientific method. At least since Karl Marx penned his famous "Theses on Feuerbach," critical theorists have taken issue with the presumption to pure theoretical reflection devoid of historical influence or practical interests. Marx insisted that scientific theorizing does much more than ethereally reflect on the nature of reality. It is, for better or worse, a product, feature, and consequential producer of reality. Hence, for most Marxian critical theorists, the idea that knowledge could ever be "detached" or "disinterested" is at best a mistake and at worst a ruse designed to mask the complicity of intellectual authority with political and economic power.

The ideas that reason and knowledge are not detached and disinterested but historically conditioned and materially embodied forms of practical engagement with the world are also central to another influential form of critical theory, American pragmatism. The pragmatists argued that knowledge production, scientific or otherwise, should be freed from the misconceived dream of transcending the human condition. Epistemic standards should instead reflect our much more realistic concerns to merely improve the human condition. By pragmatist lights, scientific theorizing consists not in developing what the philosopher Richard Rorty (1979) called a mirror of nature but in developing habits and practical skills that promote the good of the individual and society. Moreover, grounded as they are in the pursuits of actual communities, our theories and the epistemic standards by which they are evaluated are best understood with reference to the interests and activities of those for whom they hold rather than as abstract, universally valid principles. Pragmatists advise us to expect our epistemic terms of reference to be multiple and to change along with the changing conditions under which they are applied. The comparative evaluation of competing knowledge claims is not forsaken but nested deeply within the specific practical contexts within which it must inevitably be accomplished.

It is only under the specific conditions of their practical use that we may judge the adequacy of our theories, the standards by which they are judged, or the adequacy with which they have been applied in any given case. Insofar as our theories and epistemic standards are devised, learned, and applied in the course of specific practical activities, it follows that, in the first instance, those theories and standards are tied to those activities rather than the particular people who participate in them. Whereas philosophically foundationalist epistemologies have tended to cast knowing as a relationship between an isolated rational mind (or linguistic proposition) and an enduring and self-consistent natural world, critical theorists with an interest in praxis tend to cast knowing as a matter of observably competent performance within a particular domain of practical activity. Epistemic standards cease to be seen as fixed universal rules for linking "the mind" or "language" with a preformed natural world and come instead to be seen as provisional and socially situated rules for defining and identifying degrees of performative excellence.

Because their valid definition, identification, and practical engagement are inevitably predicated on these provisional and socially situated rules, the ontological characteristics of both knowing subjects and known objects lose their fixity and universality. Whatever characteristics subjects and objects (e.g., selves and their addictions) are observed to possess are held to exist only in and through the embodied activities constituting the particular practical domains in which they are observed. This theoretical orientation suffuses all the following chapters. In chapter 4, for example, I show how the addictions held to afflict participants in three recovery programs were given empirical form and causal force only in and through the distinctive patterns of therapeutic practice found in these programs. Participants' addictions were often identified and engaged in ways that bore no evident relationship to formally codified nosologies like the *Diagnostic and Statistical Manual of Mental Disorders* (DSM) of the American Psychiatric Association, and assessments of both their presence and absence in people's behavior were dictated only by the moral economy of program practice. Genetic, neurological, and other kinds of biomedical theories and evidence that might be used to great advantage in other recovery settings had absolutely no part in it. This is not to argue that ontology ought to be reduced to epistemology. Rather, it is to argue that neither our various ontologies nor our various epistemologies should be divorced from the historically situated social practices within which they arise, develop, and are given meaning and value.

Subjectivism and Objectivism

At least since René Descartes decisively cleaved *res cogitans* from *res extensa*, Western intellectuals have felt a strong compulsion to categorically distinguish the ontology of subjectivity from the ontology of objectivity. For Descartes, epistemic certainty was attained through the withdrawal of our reflections from both tradition and the evidence of our senses. Because both of these sources of information are capable of deceiving us, the achievement of genuinely valid knowledge required a skeptical introversion into a realm of purely subjective critical reflection. Following Descartes's conceptual disengagement of mind from body, the next major philosophical statement concerning the relation between subjectivity and objectivity was produced by John Locke. Locke effectively inverted Descartes's privatization of epistemic legitimacy by casting the human mind as at birth a tabula rasa, or blank slate, that acquired valid knowledge only through public dialogue concerning the evidence of our senses. While intrinsically fallible, the public tribunal of reason was nonetheless for Locke the most credible source of valid beliefs.

Locke's fallibilism has not sat well with a number of Western philosophers and scientists who have sought a more intellectually decisive procedure for separating fact from fiction. Beginning with Immanuel Kant, philosophers have long sought to overcome the apparently intransigent problem of producing objective truth claims that are invulnerable to the cacophony of public debate. This is certainly true of most addiction scientists. For his part, Kant sought to show that philosophy could produce a system of purely logical propositions that are true by definition (e.g., all bachelors are unmarried) rather than empirical, or true by virtue of their relation to the objective world (e.g., all men are mortal). To the extent science trades primarily in producing the latter form of claim, it is vulnerable to being disproved on the basis of new empirical evidence. Following Kant, many philosophers have claimed that because logic is not contingent on the available empirical evidence, it can provide universally valid guidance as to both the basic requirements any sound investigation will entail (e.g., rules of statistical inference) and what it is reasonable to seek to discover (e.g., natural laws rather than ethical facts). This project was also heavily influenced in the twentieth century by the logical positivists.

Unfortunately, though, while these schools of thought provide procedural imperatives for research, they nonetheless remain reliant on categorical distinctions between the ontology of subjectivity and the ontology of objectivity. The ontology of the objective world is cast as mind-independent and therefore demands that we somehow forge an adequate epistemological bridge between subjective perception and belief, on the one hand, and a mind-independent objective universe on the other. Because they have radically severed questions of epistemology from questions of ontology, those who have followed in the Kantian tradition have ultimately rendered the ontologically real epistemologically unknowable. The critical theoretical traditions I have followed reject this subject/object antinomy in favor of an ontology of emergent collective practice. According to these traditions, the ontology of objectivity is conceived in intersubjectively practical terms as the worlds we produce and/or discover together—that is, invariably through the activities we share with other members of particular cohorts. This understanding of the relationship between subjectivity and objectivity suffuses the following chapters.

In place of the metaphysical chasm Kantians have posited between a putatively mind-independent objective reality and subjective, including scientific, perception and agency is inserted the perceptual habits Harold Garfinkel held constitutive of what he called the natural attitude. Habit indispensably furnishes a pretheoretical empirical world of perceptible ontological topics irreducible to the analytic resources we use to theoretically account for them. It is therefore prospectively useful to discursive knowledge production in a way that a mind-independent world, because it is by definition unperceived, can never be.[1] As the acclaimed historian of science Lorraine Daston (2008, 99) has argued, "It is habit that makes perception of a world possible.... The novice sees only blurs and blobs under the microscope; experience and training are required in order to make sense of this visual chaos, in order to be able to see *things*." Citing the biologist Ludwik Fleck's groundbreaking contributions to our understanding of the ontology of disease, Daston (2008, 100) writes,

> For Fleck, learning to see like a scientist was a matter of accumulated experience—not only of an individual but of a well trained collective. The fault line in epistemology did not run between subjects and objects, the great Kantian divide, but, rather, between inexperience and experience. Unlike the neo-Kantians, who worried about how the subjective mind could know the objective world, Fleck was concerned with how perception forged stable kinds out of confused sensations.... Another way of putting this contrast is to say that Fleck was more interested in ontology than in epistemology.

Fleck's attention to the collective orchestration of perceptual habit formation predates Garfinkel's inauguration of ethnomethodology but resonates deeply with ethnomethodology's attention to the collective orchestration of the tacit, taken-for-granted competences constitutive of what ethnomethodologists call membership. It should also be emphasized that by foregrounding members' regard for one another's observable competencies rather than the tacit perceptual habits these observed competencies reveal, neither Fleck nor ethnomethodologists need to view different members' tacit competences as identical to one another. While it may be sensible to endorse Garfinkel's observation that the intrinsic accountability of practical action fosters the acquisition and habituation of capacities to competently participate in shared practices, we need not assume these tacit capacities, or habits, take identical forms (S. Turner 1994). These practical and perceptual habits need only be sufficiently attuned to allow for meaningful collaboration. Disagreement over the ontological character of what we perceive under microscopes or otherwise remains, despite our differences, a form of meaningful collaboration.

Micro and Macro

It has long been broadly held that whereas macro levels of analysis invoke structural causes of both large- and small-scale social action, micro levels of analysis drill down to consider the granular details of social interaction, largely sidestepping structural causes in their explanations and instead looking at social action as a negotiated process undertaken among subjective agents. Even among proponents of the brain disease paradigm, it is growing increasingly common to see acknowledgments of the importance of macro social variables like poverty, marginality, racism, homophobia, social cohesion, or community as important predictors of both the onset of addictions and recovery from them. These kinds of variables have long been the bread and butter of social scientific studies of addiction (Alexander 2008; Bourgois and Schonberg 2009; H. Levine 1978; Waterston 1993).

For example, as is explored in detail in chapter 2, both the historical and ethnographic literatures on drug and alcohol use have vastly enriched our acquaintance with the lived experience of drug use and addiction, and the extent to which it is inextricably entwined with broader economic, political, and cultural realities. However, as I argue throughout this book, this literature is considerably more silent as to how precisely we might best conceptualize addiction as a loss of self-control. Largely devoted to describing how *unproblematic* drinking and drug use can be interpreted as adaptive to local structural circumstances, this literature tends to overlook the sometimes seemingly self-destructive addictive aspects of drug and alcohol use (Douglas 1987; Heath 2012; Room 1984; Singer 2012). And most work specifically focused on addiction itself tends to foreground language and social structural deprivation. Some ethnographies suggest that addiction discourse be understood as what C. Wright Mills (1940) famously called "vocabularies of motive" furnished by, for example, addiction treatment clinics (Carr 2011; Davies 1992; Garcia 2010; Weinberg 2000a), while others highlight that putative addictions are often practical adaptations to the hardships of social structural deprivation and oppression (Bourgois and Schonberg 2009; Garcia 2010; Waterston 1993; Weinberg 2005). These studies vividly demonstrate the macro structural and cultural conditions under which people make their micro-level decisions about drug use, addiction, and recovery but rarely, if ever, explicitly consider the question of whether and how addiction reflects a loss of self-control.

While these insights valuably encourage more attention to how addictions can be remedied through social structural interventions, it is less obvious how they mitigate putative addicts' ethical accountability for their specific responses to the deprivations and oppressions they suffer. However, as is argued throughout this book, a therapeutic frame for addiction requires that we interpret putative addicts as somehow afflicted and therefore in need of care. Hence, warranting and implementing a therapeutic frame for addiction does not in the first instance require theories that serve only to explain the general causes of putatively addicted behaviors; it specifically requires theories that allow these behaviors to be, at least partially, ethically disowned. It is only by distinguishing the free agency of addicts' particular selves, their self-control, from the causal effects of their specific addictions that people might be simultaneously understood as amenable to therapeutic empowerment or emancipation from their addictions through recovery and somehow also afflicted by an addiction that justifies and demands such a therapeutic engagement in the first place.

Presentism and Historicism

The history and sociology of science are often framed with respect to whether they are presentist, historicist, or some combination of both. Presentist research with respect to both past and contemporary science is said to be largely extractive. That is, by presentist lights, science is read for its contributions, or lack thereof, to presently valued debates largely without reference to the biographical, intellectual, and social contexts that gave rise to its production. By contrast, historicist research is precisely concerned to situate science within the various biographical, institutional, cultural, economic, and moral contexts within which it was produced and to which its authors and audiences were at the time oriented and accountable. Over the past several decades, orthodox presentist research has been much maligned in the history and sociology of science. It is said to be Whiggish, teleological, or mistakenly devoted to the idea that science develops in a linear and progressive direction wherein the past must be judged as nothing more than a repository of preliminary successes and failures to achieve what we are now more successful in achieving. Historicists complain that not only is this approach hopelessly naive and inadequate to the task of providing for the actual historical evolution of science, but it also neglects the extent to which history, taken on its own terms rather than our own, can provide a wealth of resources with which to improve and enrich present science.

Science, both good and bad, is invariably marked by the moral and cultural climates within which it is conducted. However, due primarily to the moral and cultural climate within which addiction science is currently conducted, many of us have too often lost sight of this. Instead of understanding current science within, and in light of, its moral and cultural contexts, many of us have sought more to extricate addiction science from its locations in history and to provide, in the words of Pierre Bourdieu (2004, 1), "trans-historical truths, independent of history, detached from all bonds with both place and time and therefore eternally and universally valid." Contra Bourdieu's aspirations, my own work has been consistently and resolutely opposed to the idea that science might be productively cleansed of its historicity.

However, this has not meant that I have sought to relinquish a claim to objectivity or a commitment to scientific progress in the present. My own view is that present debate can often be improved on by a greater critical historical appreciation of precisely how and why particular theoretical positions have variously gained ascendancy in both the past and the present. For example, in addiction science we must ask not only of the logical and evidentiary grounds supporting different theories but also what broader political and cultural factors have encouraged greater and lesser attention to the needs of addicts or their respective communities over time, or the political and cultural factors that encouraged optimism or pessimism regarding recovery from addiction. Such inquiry often serves to fruitfully remind us that without exception science is embedded in, and necessarily responsive to, complex and multivalent historical contexts that extend well beyond the demands of logic and empiricism (Jasanoff 2011; Longino 2002; Rouse 2002). Perhaps even more valuably, it serves to illuminate in critical and sociohistorical terms just how present debate has arrived at where it has.

Some Last Remarks

As readers might already have inferred, I disagree with those who suggest that history, ethnography, and critical theory are independent and autonomous intellectual pursuits bearing only occasional relevance to one another. In the mid-twentieth century, it was routine to distinguish narratives concerning particular elements of the past from narratives concerning particular cultures, subcultures, or institutions in the present and to distinguish both from theoretical narratives focused on the universal and enduring nature of society as such. Moreover, moral philosophy and theories of justice were also cast in universal terms that typically underappreciated the importance of particular historical and ethnographic contexts, or what Wittgenstein called "forms of life," to the adequate defense of theories of the good and the just (Calhoun 1995; Laidlaw 2014).

I have instead followed the Marxian and pragmatist traditions in collapsing the theory/practice dichotomy and rendered theory (or theorizing) as a particular species of worldly and embodied practical action. Likewise, I have rejected one-sided determinist explanations that cast the practices available to ethnographic observation as mere epiphenomena of macro-structural dynamics like capitalism or institutionalized racism. As I have said, such reductions beg the question of our specific ethical accountabilities for the ways in which we have sought to contend with these macro-structural dynamics or, for that matter, with each other. Conversely, though, it is equally untenable to presume that collectively orchestrated social practices can be adequately understood without attention to the inequalities of power reproduced through macro-structural dynamics. Hence, I have sought to bring history, ethnography, and critical theory together as integrated facets of a holistic critical social science, always mutually implicative of one another in a variety of important ways.

Likewise, I have rejected the categorical distinction between the social and the clinical sciences. Many in addiction science categorically distinguish addiction medicine (as the clinical application of biomedical, largely neurological understandings of the nature and etiology of addiction) and the social scientific study of addiction (as the investigation of environments that foster addiction, recovery, or discourses thereof). As noted earlier, this stems largely from the overwhelming tendency in addiction science to conceptualize human biology and human social life dichotomously as two, and only two, wholly discrete and independently integrated ontological domains. One can see this dichotomy throughout the addiction sciences but it is particularly vividly exemplified in the neurological tendency to distinguish primary from secondary reinforcers of drug-using behavior, as is discussed in detail in chapter 6.

The Chapters in Brief

Chapter 1 provides a critical survey of sociological research on addiction. It begins with the seminal research of Alfred Lindesmith on heroin addiction and then proceeds through discussions of functionalist contributions, research that exemplifies what David Matza (1969) called the "appreciative" turn in the sociology of deviance, rational choice theories, and social constructionist approaches. It is confined to research on addiction in its original meaning as putative enslavement to a substance or activity rather than merely deviant or disapproved activity more broadly. As will be seen, though, there is a ubiquitous and theoretically interesting tendency even among those who contend to be writing about addiction to slip into modes of analysis that effectively substitute questions regarding the social approval of an activity for questions concerning whether it is voluntary or involuntary. Hence, one purpose of this chapter is to begin to explore whether, and how, this slippage might be avoided.

As I noted previously, mainstream addiction science is at present widely marked by an antinomy between a neurologically determinist understanding of the human brain "hijacked" by the biochemical allure of intoxicants and a liberal voluntarist conception of drug use as a free exercise of choice. Chapter 2 contrasts these two contemporary discourses to two others that played vital historical roles in initiating both scientific and popular concern for addiction. These are the Puritan and civic republican discourses that dominated scholarly discussions of addiction in the early modern era. By comparing them to their early modern historical antecedents, this chapter seeks to reflexively explore and develop more intellectually sound and therapeutically relevant alternatives to the troubled attempts at universality and value neutrality now fettering debates in mainstream addiction science.

In chapter 3, the evolution of Alfred Lindesmith's classic theory of addiction is analyzed as a product of the particular intellectual currents and controversies in and for which it was developed. These include the conflicts that pitted qualitative against quantitative sociology; the discipline of sociology against medicine, psychiatry, and psychology; and advocates of therapy for addicts against those who would simply punish them. By casting the meaningful experience of drug effects exclusively in terms of symbolically mediated mental representations of brute physiological sensations, Lindesmith's theory posits an untenable dualism between mental and bodily perception that unnecessarily limits the explanatory scope of sociological research. As an alternative to this dualism, a praxiological approach to the meaning of drug-induced behavior and experience is proposed.

A growing trend in social research concerning illicit drug use has entailed suspending regard for conventional questions such as the etiology of drug problems and the outcomes achieved by assorted interventions in favor of focusing analytic attention on how drug problems are socially constructed in and through human praxis. In chapter 4, I use a constructionist approach to ethnographically demonstrate and explain endogenous accounts of what I am calling the ecology of addiction in drug abuse treatment discourse. These accounts posit a space "out there" marked by its degradation, dirtiness, solitude, and savagery that commonly tempts those who must live there to also behave amorally, licentiously, and/or savagely. I explain these accounts by showing their fundamental utility in light of specific conceptual puzzles that participants in drug abuse treatment discourse must inevitably solve. Namely, speaking in terms of this ecology of addiction provides participants with a compelling narrative means for reconciling the following two claims: (1) they are chronically prone to enslavement by their addictions and (2) their addictions can be controlled through ongoing participation in a communal project of mutual help.

In chapter 5, I consider the value of interpreting addiction as a form of weakness of the will and/or akrasia. I then consider three problems that arise from adopting the specific views defended by those who have explicitly made the case for this thesis as well as some of their less explicit fellow travelers. The first problem is that this thesis too often posits the rational unity of properly functioning or healthy self-control as an integrated source of evaluation and volition. There are very good reasons to believe to the contrary, though, that properly functioning healthy people exhibit varying degrees of rational unity and disunity that are often explicable sociologically. The second problem is that this thesis too often posits self-control as invariably an exercise in emotional restraint, response inhibition, or delayed gratification. Once again, however, there are very good reasons to believe self-control is also exercised through self-discovery and self-actualization, which are not so obviously opposed to emotional expression, disinhibition, and personal gratification. Finally, the addiction as akrasia thesis tends to undertheorize the intrinsic relationship between experience, evaluation, and volition and the social contexts within which these are shaped, stabilized, stimulated, and sustained. Chapter 5 concludes with some brief reflections on the ramifications of these arguments for addiction science and treatment.

Chapter 6 argues that, while social contexts have long been understood to play an important role in addiction and recovery, the mechanisms through which contexts are currently said to influence addictive behavior are invariably cast as mere cues, "secondary reinforcers," or as diverse types of incentives and disincentives that induce addictive behavior. As a result, addiction is cast as either a fundamentally neurological matter with only ancillary and arbitrary links to social context or as the product of social contextually informed cost-benefit analyses. As is shown, in both cases addiction is ultimately construed as essentially a harmful and recurrent yearning for immediate self-gratification. But if indeed this is the essence of addiction, then on what grounds shall we argue that addicts are in need, and deserving, of compassion and therapy as opposed to mere disincentives or punishment?

Drawing on Foucault's work on practices of freedom and Bourdieu's notion of habitus, chapter 6 describes one particularly robust way that the influence of social context on addiction can be explained without thereby weakening the warrant for therapeutic care.

The core criterion of addiction is the loss of self-control. Ironically enough, however, neither the social nor the biomedical sciences of addiction have so far made any measurable headway in linking drug use to a loss of self-control. In chapter 7, I begin by demonstrating the limitations in this regard suffered by the social and biomedical sciences. Whereas the social sciences have variously reduced addicted drug use to deviant but nonetheless self-governed behavior or discourses thereof, the biomedical sciences have failed to adequately specify, let alone empirically analyze, how we might distinguish addicted from self-governed behavior. I then show how these limitations can be very easily overcome by the adoption of a posthumanist perspective on self-control and the various afflictions, including addiction, to which it is regarded heir. This argument provides occasion to acquaint readers with posthumanist scholarship concerning a spectrum of relevant topics, including the human body, disease, drug use, and therapeutic intervention, and to show how these lines of investigation combine to provide an innovative, theoretically robust, and practically valuable method for advancing the scientific study of addiction specifically as the loss of self-control. The chapter concludes with a discussion of some of the more important ramifications that follow from the adoption of a posthumanist approach for drug-policy studies.

SOCIOLOGICAL PERSPECTIVES
ON ADDICTION

In sociology, addiction has been approached from several distinct theoretical vantage points. Regrettably, the term has often been used interchangeably with other terms, including deviant drug use, drug misuse, and drug abuse.[1] Such imprecision results in a confusion of questions concerning the social approval of various sorts of drug use, with questions concerning whether this use is voluntary. Much of the history of social policy concerning psychoactive drugs has been predicated, at least ostensibly, on the claim that these substances possess unusual powers over people and must be regulated to protect citizens from their own personal proclivities to succumb to addictive use. If we are not able to distinguish claims regarding the putative morality of drug use from claims regarding people's ability to control their use, we are poorly equipped to effectively evaluate the history of policies predicated on the notion that people need protection from putatively addictive substances. We are also poorly equipped to evaluate social research that either endorses or rejects this idea. If it is to have any meaning at all, the term *addiction* cannot be considered synonymous with terms denoting voluntary drug use.[2]

This chapter will be confined to research that speaks to addiction as such rather than disapproved drug use more broadly. As will be seen, though, there is a ubiquitous and theoretically interesting tendency even among those who contend to be writing about addiction to slip into modes of analysis that effectively substitute questions regarding the social approval of drug use for questions concerning whether it is voluntary or involuntary. Hence, one purpose of this chapter is to explore whether, and how, this slippage might be avoided. The chapter is divided into five sections. The following section outlines and critically evaluates the seminal contributions of Alfred Lindesmith to the sociology of addiction. Next, I address the work of major functionalists who have sought to theorize addiction. I then consider the various perspectives on addiction developed by those who exemplify what David Matza (1969) dubbed the "appreciative" tradition in the sociology of deviance. In the following section, I consider the efforts of theorists who have sought to subsume addiction into the rational choice model of social action. Finally, I discuss the important contributions to the sociology of addiction made by social constructionists, particularly those inspired by the work of people such as Michel Foucault and Bruno Latour. I conclude with a brief statement of my own position.

Alfred Lindesmith: The Father of the Sociology of Addiction

The earliest and, by far, the most influential sociological research concerned specifically with addiction was conducted by Alfred Lindesmith (1938a, 1938b, 1940a, 1940b, 1947, 1968). More than eighty years after its original publication, his theory remains widely considered the classic sociological theory of addiction (see Akers 1992; McAuliffe and Gordon 1974; Stephens 1991). Lindesmith's groundbreaking achievement was to show that in addition to affecting the body biochemically, drugs and the experiences their ingestion produce are meaningful to people in ways that cannot be reduced to the interactions of a chemical agent with a human physiological system. Hence, above and beyond biochemistry, Lindesmith persuasively argued that to understand addiction it is indispensable to consider addicts' subjective perceptions of drugs, drug effects, and their wider social lives. Lindesmith noted that users who acquired heroin on the street were often vulnerable to addictive patterns of use, but those who had been administered opiates in hospital settings were not so vulnerable. He explained this by suggesting that whereas both hospital and street users experience physiological withdrawal symptoms upon cessation of use, only street users become consciously aware of the fact that the source of their distress lies in their heroin deprivation. Lindesmith argued that by using drugs specifically to alleviate withdrawal, mere drug users were transformed into genuine drug addicts.

While Lindesmith's theory retains its canonical importance, it has been subject to several serious critiques. As chapter 3 shows in detail, his theory relies on an outdated division of human perception into (1) brute biological sensations the body passively experiences in immediate response to its physical environment and (2) the mind's active and deliberate interpretation of those sensations. This voluntaristic understanding of meaning and interpretation profoundly undermines Lindesmith's capacity to theorize addiction as a loss of self-control or as something suffered rather than chosen. Moreover, Lindesmith also presumes that physiological withdrawal distress is a necessary prerequisite for the onset of addictive behavior. But the era has now passed when people could speak confidently of a distinction between drugs that produce genuine, or *physical*, addictions and drugs that produce only a more nebulous *psychological* addiction. The single most important catalyst to this era's passing was the advent of crack. Crack cocaine is widely recognized as extremely addictive by clinical professionals and nonprofessionals alike, but, oddly enough, it produces no gross physiological withdrawal symptoms (Gawin 1991).[3] The same can also be said of nicotine and all the so-called behavioral addictions, such as sex, gambling, eating, et cetera.

Furthermore, Lindesmith's reliance on the distinction between physical and psychological addiction always suffered another serious analytic problem: relapse. Many consider relapse, or the resumption of a dispreferred pattern of behavior despite one's desire not to, as the defining mark of addiction. Theories that trade on the distinction between genuine physical addiction and a less severe psychological addiction cannot remain consistent in their explanations of relapse. Lindesmith (1968, 154) explained the resumption of drug use after withdrawal symptoms have ceased primarily in terms of the former addict's subconscious generalization of the response to withdrawal distress to other forms of stress. This theory is plainly residual in the sense that it pastes a new subconscious mechanism onto the original physiological withdrawal-plus-knowledge-of-withdrawal theorem. Moreover, it is not consistently supported by empirical data on opiate addiction (Robins 1993) and affords no explanation of relapse into the use of substances such as nicotine or crack, which do not produce gross physiological withdrawal symptoms in the first place. Given the analogous tendency of former crack and nicotine addicts (to say nothing of behavioral addictions like eating, gambling, and sex) to relapse, we must look beyond the generalization of withdrawal distress to adequately understand this process.

The Functionalist Input

During the mid-twentieth century, functionalist sociologists offered a variety of theories of addictive behavior that departed in important ways from Lindesmith's seminal work. Seeking more social structural explanations, these theorists shared in common a departure from Lindesmith's presumption of a necessary physiological component to addiction. But in so departing, they also slipped from analyzing addiction as a loss of self-control into analyses of merely deviant drug use.

In his famous essay "Social Structure and Anomie," Robert Merton (1938) suggested that chronic drunkards and drug addicts might exemplify the retreatist adaptation, one of his five modes of adjustment whereby people adopt ostensibly deviant patterns of action. According to Merton, addicts could be understood as people who believe in the propriety of both the cultural goals and the institutionalized procedures society affords for achieving those goals but who cannot produce the desired results by socially sanctioned means. The result is a retreat from social life into "defeatism, quietism, and resignation" (Merton 1938, 678). This proposition was further developed in the 1960s by Richard Cloward and Lloyd Ohlin (1960) in what became their influential "double failure" hypothesis regarding addictive behavior. Contra Merton, Cloward and Ohlin suggested addicts were not *opposed* to adopting illegitimate means of achieving legitimate cultural goals but were incapable of using even these means for securing social rewards. Hence, addicts were double failures in the sense that they failed to achieve by either legitimate or illegitimate means. Heavy drug use was held to alienate putative addicts from both mainstream and delinquent subcultures, thus further reducing opportunities for social success.

Some functionalists moved beyond explanations of the distribution of addicts across social structural positions to consider the social psychological processes that motivated addictive patterns of alcohol or drug use. The best known of these was "normative ambivalence theory," which argues that drinking or drug problems will result when, in a culturally heterogeneous society, agents are bombarded with competing normative orientations to the use of alcohol and/or drugs. Under such conditions, agents, be they persons or social groups, will be unable to make unequivocal recourse to a consistent normative code concerning the use of alcohol or drugs and will thus oscillate between approval and disapproval of a given pattern of drug or alcohol use.[4] In his critique of this approach, Robin Room (1976) brilliantly shows how, in the ideological and theoretical climate of mid-twentieth-century American sociology, ambivalence became a chosen theoretical commitment largely without need of supporting empirical evidence. He wrote,

> In essence, then, our argument is that, given a societal model with only two levels, the individual and the whole system, and given an assumption that norms operate only to constrain individual deviant behavior, an explanation of the occurrence and continuation of deviance which is not completely individualistic—i.e. in terms of an inherently defective deviant individual—must be made in terms of a repeated defective interaction involving the norm—an explanation for which ambivalence provides a convenient and apparently supra-individual and explanatory rubric. (Room 1976, 1053)

As Room and others have made clear, however, there are several significant difficulties with this explanatory rubric. First, it begs many questions regarding exactly how, when, and why norms come into conflict and presumes that normative conflict is necessarily a source of stress for those who do experience it. Second, it uncritically assumes human behavior is somehow directly determined by social norms, a position that has been cast in considerable doubt (Bourdieu 1990; Garfinkel 1967; Wittgenstein 1958). Furthermore, even if it is allowed that under certain clearly specified conditions normative conflict does produce stress, we are still left to explain why this stress, in its turn, produces chronically deviant, let alone involuntary, behavior. Because existing normative ambivalence theories afford us no guidance with respect to these questions, I agree with Room when he suggests a healthy skepticism regarding their value as explanations of addiction.

According to functionalists, apparently addictive behavior patterns are best regarded as eminently rational, if painful and socially notorious, adaptations to social structural conditions. Functionalist approaches tended to stereotype addicts as necessarily socially disadvantaged and to sometimes confuse the trappings of poverty with the trappings of addiction. Moreover, they remained conspicuously silent on the question of whether addictive behavior ought to be understood as involuntary or merely socially disapproved, largely forsaking attention to the former in favor of the latter. But they did have the virtue of freeing sociological research from the presumption of a brute biological basis for addiction and of allowing sociologists to entertain the possibility that people might experience drug problems simply as a result of how they had learned to *use* these substances to cope with the social structural circumstances of their lives.

As part of a broadly based turn against functionalism in the second half of the twentieth century, many sociologists began to distance themselves from what David Matza (1969), in his book *Becoming Deviant*, dubbed the "correctional" perspective often found in functionalist theories of deviant drug use and adopt what he called an "appreciative" analytic stance largely informed by ethnographic and other qualitative types of data. Noting that modern societies are much more fragmented and conflicted than functionalists had usually allowed, these researchers advocated an agnostic moral regard for putatively dysfunctional or deviant behavior and an effort to empathize with those labeled deviant. No longer was it assumed that behavior reviled by elites or the mainstream was necessarily problematic for those who themselves engaged in the behavior. Nor was it any longer assumed that the social mechanisms according to which these behaviors were produced and sustained need reflect a functional breakdown of either the individual or their society (H. Becker 1953; Preble and Casey 1969; Sutter 1966).

Instead of investigating the mechanisms of functional breakdown, qualitative sociologists of deviance turned their attentions to providing richly detailed descriptions of drug cultures (Finestone 1957; Johnson 1980; Rosenbaum 1981; Rubington 1968), the social settings of drug activity (Sutter 1969; Wiseman 1970), the ritual practices attendant to drug use in natural settings (Waldorf, Reinarman, and Murphy 1991; Williams 1992), and the self-identities of drug users (Denzin 1993; Lindesmith 1968; Ray 1961). These studies inaugurated a thriving tradition of naturalistic investigations into drug use and drug users that has vastly enriched our understanding of the meanings attendant to drugs and drug experiences for those involved in these worlds. They have thereby extended and elaborated on Lindesmith's seminal insight that drugs, and the experiences their ingestion produce, are meaningful to people in ways that cannot be reduced to the interactions of a chemical agent with a human physiological system. However, so concerned have most of these researchers been to avoid the appearance of moralism, they have often overlooked the fact that the loss of self-control over drug use is often taken seriously by drug users themselves and is not necessarily imposed from without by moral entrepreneurs or official agencies of social control. Indeed, only a small fraction of these studies actually speak explicitly to the nature of addiction itself. Furthermore, those studies that actually do broach the nature of addiction tend to render it somewhat counterintuitively and/or in ways that do not jibe well with much of the available empirical evidence (Room 1984). This is a theme I will further elaborate on in later chapters.

For now, let me point out some general theoretical reasons this came to be the case. The appreciative turn in the sociology of deviance was heavily predicated on the symbolic interactionist school of sociological thought and naturalistic or qualitative research methods. This research was, in turn, deeply embedded in intellectual conflicts both within American sociology itself and the American academy more broadly (Weinberg 2014, 137–49). These conflicts are too nuanced to be adequately rehearsed here but, in essence, they pitted those who sought explanations for human behavior in various forms of biological, psychological, and social structural determinism against those who sought a more richly detailed understanding of their research subjects' own subjective understandings of their lives and the forms of discretion they themselves exercised both individually and collectively in orchestrating the realities of their lives. Acutely aware of the extent to which appreciative, qualitative, or subjectivist approaches to social scientific research were dismissed as anecdotal, impressionistic, and unscientific by their structurally deterministic colleagues in sociology and beyond, defenders of these approaches gravitated toward programmatic, indeed axiomatic, specifications of the human condition that highlighted the universal and intrinsic importance of local cultural meaning, subjective interpretation, and self-governance to the enactment of social life.

These axiomatic postulates were explicitly intended to protect the scientific legitimacy of naturalistic social research by highlighting the roles played by meaning making and cognitive devices such as language, myths, significant symbols, cultures and subcultures, webs of significance, or, in Norman Denzin's (1993) case, lay theories, in the production and reproduction of social structures. However, by insisting that between environmental stimulus and human behavioral response there must always be a self-governed act of meaningful interpretation, this approach to sociology made it virtually impossible to empirically study the movements into and out of self-governance that are widely held to be the defining characteristic of addictions. The emphasis placed on issues of language and cognition also tended to deemphasize the need for explicit empirical attention to the embodied practical activities in and for which these meaning-making and cognitive devices are devised and put to use. As will be seen throughout this book, the praxiological program of research I have sought to develop has been fundamentally intended to remedy these shortcomings.

I have argued that neither functionalist nor symbolic interactionist theorists have managed to avoid the implication that addictive behavior reflects a conscious, deliberate, self-governed, quasi-rational, and hence voluntary choice to use drugs. Some economists, sociologists, social psychologists, and philosophers actively embrace this position (Heather et al. 2022). While rational choice theory has contributed very few genuinely new insights into the mechanisms governing addicted behavior and has been criticized for both its rigid formalism and its inconsistency with the empirical facts (Rojeberg 2004; West 2006), it has nonetheless served to clarify the argument that addiction manifests nothing other than the cost-benefit calculations of putative addicts.

Micro-economic theorizing on addiction was inaugurated in earnest by Gary Becker and Kevin Murphy (1988), who argued that addictive behavior reflects a choice made in full knowledge of its future costs and benefits and simply reflects actors' preferences and their wider assessments of their circumstances. Most controversially, Becker and Murphy (1988) argued that actors' preferences remain stable over time and that while it may entail severe costs, this behavior is assessed by the putatively addicted actor as the best among their possible alternatives. As Athanasios Orphanides and David Zervos (1995) point out, this model yields a picture of the addict without regret and, because they already enjoy perfect foresight, beyond the reach of any instruction as to the dangers of the addicted path. Orphanides and Zervos (1995) seek to remedy this consequence by denying that the addicted actor is fully aware of the consequences of embarking on this path. While introducing the possibilities of learning, regret, and inadvertently falling into addiction, this is all predicated on the initial ignorance of the actor as to the outcome of their initiating a potentially addictive course of behavior rather than inconsistent preferences or a failure of rationality.

Others have suggested that the assumption of consistent preferences cannot be sustained in the case of addiction. Instead, they have introduced a model of the addict as prone not only to prefer present to future rewards in a consistent pattern but also to "hyperbolically discount" the prospects of future costs and benefits (Ainslie 1992). Essentially, this means we should think of human actors not as fully future-oriented cost-benefit analysts but as often vulnerable to temptations against their better judgments. The greater the prospect of immediate reward and the greater the expected intensity of that reward, the harder we find it to remain attentive to our longer-term plans. This approach forsakes the orthodox rational choice model, recasting cost-benefit calculation so as to better accommodate the fact that costs and benefits are often valued very differently, depending on their perceived imminence. Others associated with choice theory have sought to better attune considerations of cost-benefit calculation to both its external environmental cue, and internal visceral impulse, sensitivity (Elster 1999).

Most now agree that the argument that addictive behavior is consistent with the axioms of orthodox rational choice theory is not very credible. While modifications to the orthodox theory have marginally increased the credibility of choice theoretic arguments, even modified arguments remain tenuously grounded in empirical data and have been criticized for merely providing formal descriptions of idealized narratives of addiction rather than explaining actual empirical instances of it (Rojeberg 2004). While it has offered little in the way of positive insight, by explicitly formalizing the thesis that addictive behavior is the product of rational and voluntary cost-benefit calculations, this tradition has served to draw into relief the stark difficulties that remain more tacit in other social scientific traditions that have construed addictive behavior as more or less deliberate and self-governed. In my view, it is in this light that the broader analytic benefits of this literature are most properly construed.

Social Constructionist Contributions

In one sense, all social scientific contributions to our understanding of addiction are social constructionist insofar as they seek to identify social forces that influence the emergence and assessment of behavior deemed addictive. In this section, however, I confine my attention to studies that seek, more radically, to argue that addiction is not only influenced by social factors but is also fundamentally a culture-bound phenomenon—that it is unintelligible outside the nexus of cultural practices and beliefs within which it is found (Keane 2002; Reinarman 2005; Room 1985; Rudy 1986; Schneider 1978; Weinberg 2005; Wiener 1981). Harry Levine (1978), for example, argues that the rise of the temperance movement reflected a larger cultural revolution that demanded heightened levels of self-control, individualism, and accountability to the demands of a capitalist economy, all of which were found incompatible with certain patterns of heavy alcohol use. Hence, the political, economic, and cultural changes that comprised the transition to modernity provided the context in which temperance ideology, and in particular the notion of addiction, could take root and appear reasonable to large numbers of people (Alexander 2008; Ferentzy 2002; O'Malley and Valverde 2004; Reinarman

2005; Reith 2019; Valverde 1998).[5] Immensely valuable social constructionist studies have also been published on the activities and influence of science in the modern history of addiction (Acker 2002; Campbell 2007; Gomart 2002; Hellman et al. 2022). Other social constructionists have looked at the role played by the criminal justice system in giving shape to not only the contemporary status of addiction as a concept but also the lives of those identified as addicts (Duster 1970; Lindesmith 1965a; Reinarman and Levine 1997). These studies highlight the importance of acknowledging that the concept of addiction has very often been used to legitimate the stigmatization, marginalization, and persecution of drug users whether or not they have lost control of their drug use. Such studies leave little doubt that criminalization has itself caused the lion's share of suffering now associated with drug use. However, they rarely if ever speak to the question of whether some drug users sometimes do in fact lose control of their drug use, let alone how this might be best understood sociologically.

Some social constructionist studies of addiction approach the phenomenon from a less historical and more ethnographic and/or biographical perspective. Based on one of the most incisive and richly nuanced studies ever conducted with cocaine users and quitters, Dan Waldorf, Craig Reinarman, and Sheigla Murphy (1991, 10) show that problematic patterns of drug use as well as difficulties quitting are overwhelmingly associated with those who lack what they call a "stake in conventional life." People who have something to lose tend to mitigate the damage drug use introduces into their lives better than those who do not. As crucial as this insight remains, it begs the question of whether addiction ought to be construed as simple bad judgment fostered by difficult circumstances or as a kind of syndrome, something seemingly more alien to us than our own faculties of judgment and by which it is possible to feel genuinely afflicted. Though I think both scenarios do occur, I don't think the former warrants the label "loss of self-control." Therefore, to the extent we wish to theorize how a learned pattern of behavior can emerge into a syndrome over which we feel little if any direct control (and by which we can experience affliction), we need a theoretical framework that does not necessarily reduce all learned behavior to a singular faculty of judgment, subjectivity, or self.

As I will demonstrate throughout this book, just such a framework is provided by the posthumanist tradition of social research. The humanist tradition pervades Western thought as it pertains to politics, morality, law, and art and is very clearly evident throughout the sociological research on addiction that I have considered here. Adherents to the humanist tradition tend to embrace an axiomatic commitment to the principle that the irreducible atoms of social life must inevitably consist only of human subjects—integrated, intentional, deliberative agents possessing interests and investments in cultural frameworks that endow their worlds with meaning, value, and distinctive rationalities. Posthumanists worry that, among other things, this imagery reifies human nature and neglects the extent to which scientific studies of primates, cyborg technologies, and artificial intelligence modify what it means to be human and indeed encourage the deconstruction of decisive conceptual boundaries between the human and the nonhuman (Haraway 1991; Hayles 1999). Others suggest that whatever humans might be, our conceptual and practical regard for them is not fixed but intimately tied to the specific networks of interacting entities, both human and nonhuman, that provide for their substantive stabilities and accountabilities (Callon 1986; Knorr-Cetina 1997; Latour 1996; Pickering 1995). Finally, because they eschew axiomatic conceptual commitments regarding the essential identity of anything, including human subjects or selves, posthumanists advise studying situated practical action directly for clues as to how identifiable things are forged, sustained, modified, fragmented, influential, or forgotten in any actual case.

As readers of this book will discover, I have found these ideas profoundly instructive in my own research on addiction. Quite unlike the largely rationalized depictions of addicted behavior we find in most social scientific research on addiction, the people I studied did not uniformly depict addiction as a self-governed activity but often characterized it as a deeply troubling and mysterious loss of self-control.[6] Well-known writers on addiction such as Stanton Peele (1989) and John Davies (1992), among others, have acknowledged such accounts are ubiquitous but suggest they are not valid descriptions of addiction but merely socially functional for those who provide and/or believe them. They note that because they must have been learned from watching others give them, these kinds of accounts must inevitably reflect the speaker's "vocabularies of motive" (Mills 1940) rather than a genuine loss of self-control. I do not dispute the claim that these accounts are functional or that they reflect conceptual commitments prevalent in the cultures to which putative addicts belong. What I do dispute is the presumption that either of these things necessarily forecloses on an account being also descriptively valid (Gubrium and Holstein 2009; Haraway 1991).

All accounts implicate their authors' extant conceptual commitments and the uses to which their authors are putting those accounts. However, that does not mean we cannot study how our research subjects collectively assess the extent to which they are supported by empirical evidence. Moreover, the radical reduction of such accounts to mere expressions of people's preconceptions and/or their instrumental interests in providing them fails to explain either the phenomenology of addiction as a source of suffering or the ways in which addictions manifest as consequential nonhuman agents in ongoing practical action. A posthumanist understanding of addiction is eminently equipped to overcome both serious failings.

Building upon Bruno Latour's work on bodily articulation, Emilie Gomart (2002, 2004) has done much to bring the insights of posthumanism to bear on the study of addiction. She takes issue with the liberal philosophical antinomy between the human subject as absolutely free and the human body as mechanically determined, conceptualizing drug use and addiction as vehicles for the articulation of human subjectivities rather than inevitably destructive of them. Gomart and Antoine Hennion (1999) fruitfully compare drug users with music aficionados to draw out the parallel processes through which people learn and prepare themselves to be moved by drugs or by music. Becoming able to yield to the pleasures of drugs entails learning certain skills and subjective transformations and is decidedly not a merely passive response to biological determinism (see also H. Becker 1953, 1967; Reinarman 2013). This is quite right. Similarly, Gomart (2002, 2004) describes how in the Blue Clinic, patients were active and tactical users of drugs rather than mere victims to them. Hence, their physiological dependence on substitution drugs is characterized as a "generous constraint," a physiological constraint on their actions that allows clinic workers to simultaneously coerce/seduce drug users into adopting more stable and less risky forms of life. What is not addressed in these studies, though, and what I have been seeking to explore in my own work, is why and how addictions might become things that feel alien, cause people to suffer, and from which we might, on occasion, seek to free them.

Concluding Remarks

Unlike Gomart, I do not conceptualize addiction as a generic *relation* between the drug user's body and a psychoactive drug. I have deliberately avoided this because most drug users do not become addicted and, as Gomart suggests, to characterize the behavior of addicts as mechanically determined by drugs themselves is empirically hopeless. Instead, following the lead of my research subjects, I conceptualize addictions as nonhuman agents residing in the bodies of those who are addicted. In opposition to biologically reductionist accounts, Latour (2004, 205) writes that "to have a body *is to learn to be affected*, meaning 'effectuated,' moved, put into motion by other entities, humans or non-humans. If you are not engaged in this learning you become insensitive, dumb, you drop dead." It is as a distinctive type of just this kind of "learn[ing] to be affected" that I want to conceptualize addictions as embodied agents. But whereas Latour (2004) appears to suggest a normative judgment that any way that bodies learn to be affected by the world should be embraced, I want to be a bit more cautious. It seems to me that to have a body is also to be vulnerable to disease (see Mol 2002; Mol and Law 2004). However, as a posthumanist, I regard diseases not merely as pathological biological mechanisms but, more generally, as patterns of *harmful* bodily articulation—that is, patterns of bodily articulation with which we cannot, or do not want to, identify ourselves precisely because they afflict or endanger those articulations with which we do self-identify. If we are clear that this is what is meant by disease, then I can see no reason to deny, and every reason to affirm, that an addiction might be just such a thing.

2

FREEDOM AND ADDICTION
IN FOUR DISCURSIVE REGISTERS
A Comparative Historical Study
of Values in Addiction Science

Mainstream addiction science is now widely, though not uniformly, marked by an antinomy between a neurologically determinist understanding of the brain "hijacked" by the biochemical allure of intoxicants and what I am calling a liberal voluntarist conception of drug use as a free exercise of choice (see Heather and Segal 2017; Heyman 2009; M. Lewis 2018; Volkow, Koob, and McLellan 2016). Prominent defenders of both discourses strive, but ultimately do not fully succeed, to provide accounts of freedom and addiction that are both universal and value neutral. This has resulted in a variety of conceptual problems and has undermined the utility of such research for those who seek to care for people presumed to suffer from addictions. In this chapter, I argue that contemporary debate would benefit substantially from a review of the discursive contexts within which the concept of addiction originally gained a degree of intellectual legitimacy and broader cultural traction. These are the Puritan and civic republican discourses that dominated scholarly discussions of addiction in the early modern era. By comparing them to their early historical antecedents, I seek to reflexively explore and develop more intellectually sound and therapeutically relevant alternatives to the troubled attempts at universality and value neutrality that now fetter debates in mainstream addiction science.

After reviewing prominent positions in the "brain disease" and liberal voluntarist discourses, I then proceed to discuss prominent positions in the early modern Puritan and civic republican discourses on addiction. In each case, the place of values in these positions is highlighted. I conclude with a statement of some of the more important ramifications that follow from a more historically informed and thereby analytically incisive understanding of the real-world vicissitudes of freedom and addiction as they take form "in the wild," to borrow Edwin Hutchins's (1995) evocative phrase—outside laboratories, and in the more therapeutically relevant contexts of people's everyday lived experiences. These ramifications include a proposed return from the present preoccupation with the dichotomy between freedom and neurological determinism to that which preoccupied early modern theorists between freedom and slavery. They also include a proposal for updating the appreciation, now lost to addiction science, that early modern theorists had for the intersection between judgments of freedom and slavery, on the one hand, and judgments of virtue and vice, on the other. This updating can be achieved by supplementing contemporary liberal theory's now preponderant tendency to equate freedom with the autonomous pursuit of hedonic values (concerning desires) with the pursuit of what Aristotle called eudaemonic values (concerning well-being).

A Note on Theory and Methodology

This chapter has been written with the intention to contribute to current debates in addiction science by recourse to early modern history. With respect, then, to the brain disease discourse and the liberal voluntarist discourse, I take constructively critical positions. These positions are predicated on my sharing a value commitment widely, but not uniformly, exhibited in these discourses to make addiction science more relevant to the work of both caring for addicts and providing broader political and cultural warrant for therapeutic care over punishment. Defenders of the brain disease paradigm have consistently emphasized the importance of defending a medical frame for drug problems not only because they believe the best neurological research suggests the scientific truth of this frame but because they believe it is culturally indispensable that we define addiction as a disease if it is to be met with enlightened societal responses, with sympathy rather than scorn (Leshner 1997). It is only thusly, they often insist, that we can argue addicts should not be blamed but helped. However, as I show, their efforts, and those of many of their most prominent critics, to foster more humane interventions are undermined by the aspirations to make universal and value-neutral scientific claims about addiction. In this chapter, I explicitly demonstrate these difficulties among both those in the disease camp and those in the liberal voluntarist camp who oppose them and seek to open a path forward through an examination of two major early modern discourses on addiction.

Hence, my analytic take on the second two discursive registers I consider is decidedly different from that I bring to bear on the first two. Rather than positioning myself as constructively critical and aligned in the project of better promoting certain values also promoted in these discourses, I take a more historicist position. In the second two cases, then, my effort is simply to reconstruct and understand the meaning these discourses had for those who participated in them without any effort to assess their validity or to improve on them by contemporary scientific lights. Instead, the purpose of these analyses is to demonstrate to readers how contemporary addiction science can better fulfill the objectives of therapeutic relevance and provide credible warrant for therapy over punishment through the selective adoption and modification of certain elements of these earlier discourses.

One reviewer of an earlier draft of this chapter usefully noted that neither determinist nor voluntarist addiction science is homogeneous and that one can, in fact, locate researchers on a continuum between determinism and voluntarism. More specifically, they proposed I stress that the following analysis makes use of Weberian ideal types to excavate and analyze how freedom and addiction are variously conceptualized in addiction science. In an important sense, this reviewer is entirely correct insofar as I do focus attention not on highlighting the diversity of positions found in addiction science but on particular major tendencies. However, as I reacquainted myself with the literature on ideal types and, in particular, the eminent Weber scholar Richard Swedberg's (2018) recent illuminating commentary, I became convinced that my own theoretical and methodological approach diverges from Weber's. For Weber, ideal types are artificial constructs, indeed fictions, with which social reality is compared. My own approach is instead to factually identify important theoretical tendencies in the addiction science literature and their ramifications with respect to our understanding of freedom and addiction. To reiterate, this study emphatically does not exhaustively catalog or comprehensively assess the neurological or social scientific literatures on addiction but is only a selective analysis of certain central and important trends.

It should also be emphasized that this analysis is focused only on demonstrating and overcoming some significant limitations that follow from the widespread efforts in both the brain disease and choice theoretic literatures to produce theories about addiction that are both universal and value free. I don't think it can be credibly denied that such research is indeed pervasive in addiction science. But this also means that to the extent contemporary research does not aspire to universality or value neutrality, it is not a central focus of my analysis. Pertinent to this point, another reviewer of an earlier draft of this chapter recommended a more thorough engagement with current anthropological research on addiction. It is certainly correct to note a long and fruitful tradition of anthropological research related to drug and alcohol use and an important flowering of ethnographic research on addiction in anthropology and allied disciplines over the past fifteen years or so (Bourgois and Schonberg 2009; Carr 2011; Dennis 2019; Dilkes-Frayne et al. 2017; Duff 2008; Fraser and Moore 2011; Garcia 2010; Gowan and Whetstone 2012; Raikhel 2016; Raikhel and Garriott 2013; Schull 2012; Weinberg 2005; Zigon 2011). This literature has vastly enriched our acquaintance with the phenomenological nuances of drug use, addiction, and the extent to which these are inextricably entwined with broader economic, political, and cultural realities.

However, it only very indirectly addresses the concerns I am raising here—that is, the limits placed on our ability in both the brain disease and liberal voluntarist literatures to produce therapeutically relevant findings or warrants for therapeutic care by the widespread scientific aspirations to produce universally valid and value-neutral theories of addiction. In fact, much of the classic ethnographic literature on drug use is both consistent with and uncritical of the universalistic and value-neutral aspirations of the liberal voluntarist discourse. This literature is largely devoted to describing the locally adopted cultural norms and practices within which *unproblematic* drinking and drug use occur rather than the sometimes seemingly self-destructive addictive aspects of their use (Douglas 1987; Heath 2012; Room 1984; Singer 2012). While culturally diverse, there is little if any suggestion that these practices are unfree. And most ethnographic work specifically focused on addiction itself tends to foreground the important roles played by language and social structural deprivation. For example, many ethnographies suggest that addiction discourse be understood as what C. Wright Mills (1940) famously called "vocabularies of motive" furnished by, for example, addiction treatment clinics (Carr 2011; Davies 1992; Garcia 2010) or that putative addictions are often practical adaptations to the hardships of social structural deprivation and oppression (Bourgois and Schonberg 2009; Garcia 2010; Waterston

1993; Weinberg 2005). These studies vividly highlight the structurally and culturally specific conditions under which people make their decisions concerning drug use, addiction, and recovery but rarely, if ever, explicitly consider the question of whether and how addiction reflects a loss of self-control.

These kinds of analyses incisively and, I would argue, crucially identify various elements of social context as integral to the production and reproduction of both addictions and discourses thereof. However, close inspection reveals they are much less explicit as to how we might warrant or inform therapeutic or exculpatory orientations to addictions. No doubt, it is certainly correct to insist that social structural dynamics powerfully encourage both putative addicts and others to construe their problems in personal rather than social structural terms and to thereby misrecognize the various ways in which those problems are caused by macro-structural regimes such as economic exploitation, racism, sexism, or homophobia (Bourgois and Schonberg 2009; Gowan and Whetstone 2012; Weinberg 2005). But while these insights valuably encourage more attention to how addictions can be remedied through social structural interventions, it is less obvious how they mitigate putative addicts' ethical accountability for their specific responses to the deprivations and oppressions they suffer. Some years ago, Erving Goffman (1961, 86–87) relevantly observed,

> Although there is . . . an environmental view of crime and counter-revolutionary activity, both freeing the offender from moral responsibility for his offence, total institutions can little afford this particular kind of determinism. Inmates must be caused to *self-direct* themselves in a manageable way, and, for this to be promoted, both desired and undesired conduct must be defined . . . as something [they] can do something about.

Goffman's observation in this regard holds not only for what he called "total institutions" devoted to the management of addictions but, indeed, wherever people wish to promote a specifically therapeutic orientation, in contrast to neurological or critical sociological orientations, to addiction—that is, to promote the emancipation of particular people from their own putative addictions rather than address addiction's general etiological causes in neurological processes, vocabularies of motive, or social oppression. However, in stark contrast to a criminalizing frame, a therapeutic frame requires that we interpret putative addicts not as culpable but as afflicted and therefore in need of care. Hence, warranting and implementing a therapeutic frame for addiction does not in the first instance require theories that serve only to explain the general causes of putatively addicted behavior; it specifically requires theories that allow these behaviors to be, at least partially, ethically disowned. It is only by distinguishing the free agency of addicts' particular selves, their self-control, from the causal effects of their specific addictions that people might be simultaneously understood as amenable to therapeutic empowerment or emancipation from their addictions through recovery and somehow also afflicted by an addiction that justifies and demands such a therapeutic engagement in the first place.

My argument is that these specifically ethical and experiential aspects of addiction and recovery have been clouded by the universalist and value-neutral aspirations observable in much of the scientific literature on addiction. These aspirations manifest, on the one hand, in neurologically and social structurally deterministic explanations that tend, as Goffman observed, to gloss the complex forms of discretion and ethical accountability that practically arise in our everyday lives, and, on the other hand, in liberal voluntarist discourses of "choice" that tend to gloss the complex ways in which our discretion and hence our individual rights and responsibilities are often practically diminished or mitigated in our everyday lives, sometimes encouraging an ethic of care over a liberal ethic of individual rights and responsibilities (see Nussbaum 2006).[1] As I have noted, universalism and value neutrality foster a tendency toward scientific and ethical detachment that is inconsistent with a therapeutic and/or ethical engagement with putative addicts' particular lived experiences. As a result, they fetter our capacities to inform or warrant the provision of therapeutic care over punishment. It is in the interest of identifying and beginning to overcome these fetters that this chapter has been written.

The Brain Disease Discourse

In a widely cited article in the *Annual Review of Neuroscience*, the distinguished neurologist Steven Hyman and his colleagues wrote, "Unlike natural rewards, addictive drugs do not serve any beneficial homeostatic or reproductive purpose but instead often prove detrimental to health and functioning. Much work over several decades has begun to paint a picture of how addictive drugs come to masquerade as, and eventually supplant, natural rewards as highly valued goals" (Hyman, Malenka, and Nestler 2006, 571).[2]

Cast in the presumptively value-neutral register of neurology, we see here an explicit contrast of natural rewards, as experiences whose value is biologically determined to foster behavior conducive to health and reproduction, with the presumptively unnatural, and health-threatening (or at least health-irrelevant), rewards of drug use. This distinction lies at the heart of the now ascendant scientific model of addiction, what historian David Courtwright (2010) has dubbed the NIDA (National Institute on Drug Abuse) brain disease paradigm. It is precisely by way of this distinction that a scientific case is made for the argument that addictive drugs deprive addicts of their freedom and thereby create a medical disability warranting medical care (Kalivas and Volkow 2005; Kelley and Berridge 2002; Robinson and Berridge 2003). By *unnaturally* "hijacking" the brain's natural proclivities to reward healthy behavior, addictive drugs deceive, usurp, and enslave the brain's reward circuitry, causing a "loss of self-control" and rendering untold harms to victims themselves and to their societies (Volkow, Koob, and McLellan 2016, 364). Ironically, there is implicit in this wholly deterministic account of the human brain and its biomechanical responses to addictive chemicals a distinct (if dubious) theory of human freedom. If addiction, or the loss of self-control, flows from our sustained indulgence in and pathological valuing of the unnatural rewards of drug use, then our freedom, or the retention of our self-control, must, by implication, consist largely in confining our attention to the value of natural, or biologically healthy, rewards.

The NIDA brain disease paradigm is undoubtedly hegemonic in contemporary addiction science but it is by no means uncontested. Critics point to the challenges of reconciling the NIDA paradigm with the epidemiological facts that only a small fraction of those who have used addictive drugs fall into detrimental patterns of use (SAMHSA 2008), that many who do fall into these patterns "mature out" of them without treatment (Robins 1993; Winick 1962), and that it is often social rather than genetic or neurological disadvantages that best predict who is most likely to succumb to addictive drug use and who is least likely to recover from it (Alexander 2008; Edwards 2005; Waldorf, Reinarman, and Murphy 1991). As awkward as these epidemiological facts certainly are for defenders of the brain disease paradigm, a still more fundamental difficulty attends their conspicuous reticence to explicitly develop their implicit orientations to freedom—that is, their views of exactly what addicts lose when they lose their self-control. However, we can begin to flesh out these views by attending to their counterparts—ascendant neurological theories of addiction itself. How do proponents of the brain disease paradigm provide for the putative loss of our freedom to addiction?

They do so in primarily two ways. First, incentive sensitization theorists argue that through sustained exposure addicts' desire (want) for drugs is neurologically disjoined from the degree to which they find pleasure in (like) drug use (Robinson and Berridge 2003). Hence, their desire for drugs is not only "unnatural" but eventually unjustified by the pleasure users believe they derive from them. This allows brain disease scientists to cast this desire as both pathological and involuntary because it is unhealthy and inconsistent with orthodox postulates of rational choice. But the equation of freedom with either health maintenance or a generic model of rationality is not scientifically sustainable. In modern liberal societies, not all unhealthy conduct, irrationality, or even misplaced desire is considered unfree, let alone pathological. In practice, people freely value a wide range of both healthy and unhealthy preferences under widely divergent conditions of (mis)understanding. Beyond valorizing health and rational choice, addiction scientists must tell us how people grow estranged from their behavior enough to warrant the claim that their self-control is genuinely afflicted, and hence their freedom attenuated, by addiction. Findings that sometimes people want things more than they like them is not sufficient warrant for such a claim.

The second way addictions are normally said to deprive people of their freedom is by compromising brain processes associated with "executive functions" (Kalivas and O'Brien 2008). These functions are not always clearly specified in the brain disease literature, but they include things such as attention, response inhibition, planning, problem solving, and working memory. Like research on incentive sensitization, this research also seeks universal and value-neutral neurological measures of freedom and addiction. But the argument that people universally equate their own or one another's freedom with long-term planning, problem solving, and impulse control is undeniably false. Not only do we freely throw caution to the wind on occasion but so too on occasion do we equate our most authentic values with our gut instincts, spontaneous desires, and other emotional impulses and, indeed, equate the kinds of cognitive processes associated with executive function with alienation from our real selves, freedom, and authentic self-control (Alasuutari 1992; Hochschild 2012; R. Turner 1976). On these accounts, our freedom is undermined rather than facilitated by the inhibitions imposed by executive functions. Indeed, a vivid and pertinent illustration of this is the extensive therapeutic emphasis drug rehabilitation programs such as Alcoholics Anonymous themselves place not on the executive repression of spontaneous emotions but on the encouragement of their free and open expression in the interest of facilitating people's better self-understanding and self-control (Carr 2011; Garriott and Raikhel 2015; Valverde 1998; Zigon 2011).

The brain disease literature's tendency to disregard the manifest diversity of empirical forms taken by freedom and addiction, self-control and its loss, stems from an evident inability or unwillingness to breach the bound-aries of brain biology in any but the most cursory manner (Campbell 2010; Vrecko 2010). While brain disease theorists allow that Pavlovian condition-ing may *arbitrarily* link environmental cues with the unnatural rewards neu-rologically intrinsic to addictive substances and activities, these are entirely ancillary to the neurological reward circuitry by which our ultimate value preferences are determined. In this way, both freedom (implicitly defined as a rational value preference for rewards conducive to biological health) and addiction (implicitly defined as an irrational value preference for rewards that may threaten health) are conceptualized as fundamentally ahistorical and neurologically determined. Addiction is thus held to afflict our personal freedom only to the extent that we equate freedom with an invariant commit-ment to value biological health above all else. While this research may very well continue to yield scientific dividends in other ways, it will never yield an empirically adequate grasp of the nuanced phenomenology of becoming es-tranged from one's own behavior—that is, losing self-control—nor the jointly intrapersonal, interpersonal, and social structural dynamics that render that estrangement so real for people. Because it fails to adequately explain the loss of self-control to addiction, this research also fails to fulfill its ethical objec-tive of providing scientific warrant for therapeutic care for addicts. Insofar as it does not fulfill its promise of distinguishing addictions, specifically as afflictions, from the free ethical agency of people who suffer from these af-flictions, brain disease discourse provides no coherent warrant for medical care over blame and punishment.

The Liberal Voluntarist Discourse

The medicalization of addiction has always been vigorously contested (Alex-ander 2008; Fraser, Moore, and Keane 2014; Granfeld and Reinarman 2015; Netherland 2012; Satel and Lilienfeld 2013). Indeed, the idea that addicts never in fact lose their freedom of choice remains widespread in both the social sciences and popular culture (Valverde 1998). Dating back at least to John Stuart Mill's essay "On Liberty" ([1859] 2005), this position has been largely based on the liberal democratic value judgments that all people should be viewed to possess the faculty of self-government and that it is unjust to suppress their free exercise thereof (Foddy and Savulescu 2010; Szasz 2003). Perhaps ironically, these value judgments have become widely entrenched in the social sciences via ostensibly value-neutral postures of agnosticism to-ward elite and/or mainstream norms disparaging historically marginalized groups and a concomitant emphasis on the local rationality of these groups and their own sense of moral legitimacy. This has been part of a more general social scientific tendency to understand social reality as invariably composed of the consensual or conflictual interactions of integrated social groups and to define their members as integrated individuals—rational, self-governing agents who affiliate with these groups based on their belief in the group's traditions, interests, or values.

Hence, more specifically, by the mid-twentieth century, putative addicts were often described as members of subcultures with their own distinctive value systems rather than sufferers of intrinsic personal afflictions or deficits of any kind (Finestone 1957; Hughes 2007; Preble and Casey 1969; Stephens 1991). Concerned about slipping from their presumed value neutrality into an illiberally biased moralism, social researchers have often overlooked the fact that addiction, understood specifically as a loss of self-control, is an idea that putative addicts often themselves take seriously and that is not necessarily coercively imposed from without. In short, social scientists have very often held that addiction reflects a notorious but nonetheless voluntary choice to value the use of drugs over matters that others in society consider more important.

Since roughly the 1980s, a growing collection of self-described "choice theorists" in sociology, economics, social psychology, philosophy, and even neuroscience itself has sought to more methodically develop this position (Davies 1992; Heather and Segal 2017; Heyman 2009; M. Lewis 2018). These theorists tend to begin with the observation that most behavior attributed to addictions is "incentive sensitive" (consistent with cost-benefit analysis) and not compulsive in the orthodox neurological sense emphasized by disease theorists. While this is true, we should not make too much of it. Plants are incentive sensitive in the sense that they grow toward resources like light and water, but we would not normally want to conceptualize this as a voluntary choice, let alone an exercise of freedom. Defending the liberal voluntarist understanding of addiction, the philosophers Bennett Foddy and Julian Savulescu (2007, 31) argue that while it may be "hopelessly romantic" to suggest that there are no biological correlates to human preferences, the reduction of freedom to the pursuit of health-relevant natural rewards is untenable. Self-government is quite obviously motivated by a wide range of values, many of which put our biological health at risk. Activities like mountaineering, refusing under torture to divulge state secrets, or even indulging a sweet tooth may very well be highly valued and freely engaged activities despite their failure to fulfill anything neurologists would regard as naturally rewarding or serving of a biologically "beneficial homeostatic or reproductive purpose" (Hyman, Malenka, and Nestler 2006, 571).

From these and similar observations, choice theorists conclude that it is scientifically false (and politically illiberal) to insist that preferences are freely adopted and natural when they foster health but unfree and unnatural when they might threaten health. Preferences, they argue, are neither natural nor unnatural. They simply reflect predispositions to avoid or relieve experiences we as individuals devalue and to pursue experiences we personally do value. And if there is no scientifically sound way to distinguish natural from unnatural preferences, there is no way of objectively distinguishing free from pathological motivations, and we must conclude that putative addicts freely choose to act as they do. According to this argument, the notion that addiction entails a loss of freedom is nothing but a myth with which we improperly exonerate people for their wrongdoings or denigrate, dehumanize, and persecute marginalized members of our societies (Davies 1992; Heather and Segal 2017; Heyman 2009; M. Lewis 2018; Szasz 2003). This argument not only flatly denies the validity of current scientific claims distinguishing addiction from freedom but, according to authors such as Foddy and Savulescu (2010), requires that any future scientific claims in this regard must be conceptualized independently of not only neurological conceptions of natural and unnatural rewards but also any substantive claims at all regarding the health or objective value of people's preferences. Citing the nineteenth-century diagnosis of "drapetomania," or the pathological propensity of slaves to run away, they write,

> In the American South during the mid-nineteenth century, it may have been difficult to believe that a sane slave would wish to escape captivity. Today, it is difficult to believe that a sane person would wish for outcomes that are harmful to their health, simply because normal people prioritize health ahead of pleasure. The case of drapetomania explains why no version of the claim that addiction is a disease should contain substantive normative claims about what a person's preferences should be. (Foddy and Savulescu 2010, 9)

Because we can find historical examples of disease categories such as drapetomania that were based on now discredited claims regarding normatively appropriate behavior, we must therefore confine the use of the concept of disease to value free and asocial accounts of biological dysfunction. While on first blush this appears plausible, there are in fact immense, and probably insurmountable, challenges to defining even physical diseases in ways that altogether avoid normative presumptions of a dispreferred state of affairs (Metzl and Kirkland 2010). This problem is particularly acute in addiction science, and indeed mental health research more generally, wherein we must contend with a much higher level of dissensus as to the natural functions and/or dysfunctions of mental structures or processes (Bolton 2010; Fulford 1989). The clinical validity of even uncontroversial psychiatric diagnoses such as obsessive compulsive disorder (OCD) or schizophrenia is invariably predicated not on generic scientific findings of biological or psychological dysfunction but on highly contingent value judgments of personal or social dysfunction furnished by patients and their significant others—that is, friends, family members, colleagues, and others with personal knowledge of the patient's unique biography and social circumstances.

On its face, one wouldn't think this should be a problem for liberal theory. After all, since its inception, liberalism has been vigorously opposed to the idea that people's values should be dictated by any singular authority, be it a king, divine will, biology, or nature more generally. It has insisted instead on a pluralistic moral universe wherein we decide for ourselves what it means to be free or to pursue our own conceptions of the good life without interference. One might reasonably expect, then, that liberal theory would also hold each of us entitled to decide if and when our freedom had been diminished and by what. But, sadly, what was once a pluralist and egalitarian ethic of moral and epistemological tolerance has for many become a presumptive social ontology wherein human behavior is axiomatically understood as always free—that is, unless physically compromised, invariably expressive of the values of its author. A prominent defender of this view, the sociologist Anthony Giddens, has insisted that someone threatened with death for defiance is still making a free choice to do as they are told, predicated on a personal value judgment that living is better than dying. In this way, only physical forces can literally determine our actions rather than merely incentivizing us, through appeals to our personal values, to freely adopt them (Giddens and Pierson 1998, 84). As the writings of Thomas Szasz and other neoliberals amply demonstrate, this ontology affords no room for *mental* disease at all. The price of its adoption is thus a dogmatic refusal to recognize any form of mental affliction that is not demonstrably linked to biological dysfunction. Because the neuroadaptations identified by brain disease theorists are not invariably dysfunctional (they result from prolonged exposure to all sources of reward), they cannot support the claim that addiction is a disease or anything other than an expression of strong but nonetheless freely pursued appetites (M. Lewis 2018).

Hence, like many contributors to the brain disease discourse, many contributors to the liberal voluntarist discourse on addiction tend to define freedom and addiction in universal and value-neutral terms. They do so not by conceptualizing freedom and addiction biologically. Instead, freedom is conceptualized a priori as an axiomatic resource with which to explain history but one that is itself a historical constant—a universal feature of human behavior that neither varies historically nor that is ever attenuated by anything other than physical constraints. While this social ontology may continue to yield other theoretical dividends, it, like the brain disease paradigm, cannot adequately provide for the nuanced phenomenology of being estranged from one's own behavior—that is, losing self-control. And, hence, to the extent they aspire to universality and value neutrality, defenders of the liberal voluntarist discourse have also provided no coherent warrant for therapeutic care as opposed to blaming addicts for their fates.

The Early Modern Puritan Discourse

Taking issue with Harry Levine's (1978) landmark analysis of the discovery of addiction, historian Jessica Warner (1994, 685) argues that the earliest exponents of the disease theory were Puritan clergyman, not physicians: "It is in the religious oratory of Stuart England that we find the key components of the idea that habitual drunkenness constitutes a progressive disease, the chief symptom of which is a loss of control over drinking behavior. By the same token, the modern conception of addiction was not, as Levine claimed, first formulated in the medical community but had previously been fulminated from the pulpit."

Warner did not take issue with Levine's distinction between addiction as sin and sickness—moral and medical orientations to addiction—but sought, instead, to insist that Levine's crediting of physicians for originating the medical concept was mistaken. This is a somewhat puzzling claim. In opposition to the distinguished medical historian Roy Porter (1985, 390), who advocated efforts to "understand the making of the idea of alcoholism within its socio-intellectual milieu, in particular in regard to changing conceptions of disease," Warner (1994, 686) argues that "the noun 'disease' appears to have had a fairly constant meaning over the past several centuries." That this argument is factually incorrect will be demonstrated later. For now, let us confine our attention to its implications for her general thesis. If religious orators in Stuart England understood the concept of disease as orthodox biomedicine does today—as a biomechanical failure of the body, involuntary and therefore morally exempt—how did they reconcile this with the traditional religious view that habitual drunkenness is a sin?

Levine (1978, 150–51) also notes cases of preindustrial clerics describing habitual drunkenness as a kind of "madness" and an "incurable" habit but argues that their Calvinist theology ultimately blocked them from accepting the idea that some forms of drinking were genuinely beyond the drinker's control.

> Puritan ministers were the most troubled by habitual drunkenness, and in some scattered phrases and sentences we find evidence of their trying to stretch beyond the ideas of their days. Increase Mather, for example, declared that habitual drunkenness was a kind of madness, and Foxcroft warned moderate drinkers that they were "in danger of contracting an incurable Habit." But the ministers were not able to synthesize their observations; they were bound by the categories of their theology and psychology . . . for Puritans. . . . The individual was always viewed as having the freedom to choose to sin or not.

Though for different reasons, Levine's argument here is also puzzling. Given their well-known doctrinal rigidity, what motivated Puritan ministers to "stretch beyond the ideas of their days"? How could Increase Mather have reconciled describing habitual drunkenness as a kind of madness with an insistence that it was nonetheless a sinful exercise of free will? Pace Levine, Warner's first attempt to solve these puzzles was to place a staunch faith in the self-evidence of experience. Puritan ministers, she argues, were not bound by their theology to interpret people's behavior as freely chosen. Their sermons were instead directly influenced by firsthand observations. After citing some instances of preachers discussing habitual drunkenness as a loss of self-control, she (1994, 688) writes, "It would be wrong to place undue emphasis on the examples just given, or to assume that the notion of addiction was central to earlier definitions of habitual drunkenness. But it would be equally wrong to assume that earlier generations were inherently incapable of describing destructive behavior in an empirical or critical fashion, or to assume that the mind-set of preindustrial society somehow blinded contemporaries to the addicts in their midst."

In this passage, Warner seems to insist that the difference between addicts and voluntary drunkards was empirically obvious and beyond debate. The Puritan clergy's theological conviction that sinful behavior invariably hailed from sinful free choices was, then, simply overwhelmed by the brute force of empirical observation. The degree of controversy that even now surrounds the very existence of addiction, let alone the diagnoses of particular cases, casts Warner's seemingly naive empiricism in considerable doubt (Alexander 2008; Reinarman 2005; Reith 2019). As we have seen, contemporary liberal theory provides robust evidence that those who choose to interpret self-destructive drinking as freely chosen behavior are quite capable of construing the empirical evidence accordingly. Hence, Warner's claim that Puritan ministers' commitment to the doctrine of free will was decisively trumped by empirical evidence alone cannot be taken seriously. Later in her article, Warner (1994, 690) proposes a second, rather more plausible, argument—that preachers' use of medical language was often just an ad hoc rhetorical strategy designed not to lay any serious claim to medical expertise but only to influence parishioners.

> We have already seen that preachers routinely cited medical evidence when exhorting their audiences to abandon the sin of drunkenness. It is perhaps in much the same spirit that friends and family might today tell a chain-smoker that he or she runs a high risk of an early death; they might say so not because they are physicians or are themselves especially familiar with the medical evidence, but because they abhor the habit in question, and knowingly resort to a variety of appeals and rhetorical stratagems in hopes of rectifying an undesirable behavior.

There is a big difference, though, between loosely invoking claims like "smoking kills" that have already been medically authorized and simply making up one's own health claims without medical authorization. If Warner is suggesting the former, her argument regarding the historical priority of the clerics' formulations is lost. If she is suggesting the latter, she must either explain what justified clerics' claims to medical knowledge independent of medical authorization or accept that their claims were not epistemologically authorized—that they were only rhetorical stratagems rather than literal descriptions. This would then beg the question of why anyone would have eventually taken such rhetoric sufficiently seriously to begin treating it literally, let alone scientifically.

Though largely critical of her analysis, Peter Ferentzy (2001, 387) agrees with Warner that clerical invocations of disease were often just ad hoc exhortations: "preachers often used terms such as 'disease' and 'sickness' loosely, with little or no suggestion that medical issues were involved." No doubt, Ferentzy is correct to advise caution in interpreting preindustrial sermons and religious commentaries too literally. It is certainly true that many religious orators had few qualms about taking rhetorical liberties or drawing upon metaphors in their efforts to sway their flocks. That said, the claim that clerical uses of medical language were never literal is empirically unsustainable. Consider the following passage on habitual drunkenness from the preeminent Puritan scholar Richard Baxter's *A Christian Directory* ([1673] 1825, 410–11):

> Had God made thee an idiot, or mad and lunatic, thy case had been to be pitied: but to make thy *self* mad and despise thy manhood, deserveth punishment. Its the saying of *Basil; Involuntary madness deserveth compassion, but voluntary madness, the sharpest whips. Judgements are prepared for scorners, and stripes for the fools back*: especially for the *voluntary fool*: He that will *make himself* a *beast* or a *mad-man*, should be used by others like a beast or a mad-man, whether he will or not.

In this passage, Baxter very clearly distinguishes divinely imposed from self-imposed madness to make a point regarding moral culpability. It is very hard to see how this could be anything other than a literal distinction. But there is a second point to be made with respect to this passage. Baxter also very clearly treats habitual drunkenness as a *sinful* madness—a madness, but one deserving of punishment. This formulation is manifestly at odds with the contemporary biomechanical formulation of disease as morally exculpatory and with the choice theoretic literature that also starkly contrasts immorality and sickness. Without impugning its contemporary ethical merits, there can be no doubt that the now scientifically entrenched categorical dichotomy between immorality and sickness is inconsistent with much of the historical record of how early modern Europeans oriented to habitual drunkenness (Baumohl and Room 1987; Nicholls 2009; Valverde 1998). It also leaves anomalous the fact that religious writers historically preceded physicians in literally asserting that habitual drunkenness is often an enslaving disease. This anomaly can be resolved by recalling the relationship people of the period routinely drew between religion and health.

During the seventeenth and eighteenth centuries, most Protestants understood all diseases as products of humanity's fall from grace and, in the case of particular communities or individuals, God's punishment of sin (Starr 1982; Thomas 1971).[3] By the eighteenth century, it was a cultural commonplace that temperate eating and drinking habits, sex lives, and lifestyles more generally were healthy because virtuous and, to some extent, virtuous because healthy.[4] The Enlightenment certainly fostered more optimism as to the possibility of proactively overcoming human ills, but this did not supplant so much as transform the putative role of God in creating, and religious virtue in stemming, those ills. God was now understood to reward virtue and punish vice less through the mysterious dictates of his divine discretion than the divinely authored medium of nature, the laws of which could be discerned and honored through use of his greatest gift to humanity—our reason. People retained their health by use of this divine gift to better understand and to more strictly obey the dictates of God's natural design.

That this fusion of religious and medical thought served as a commonsense backcloth to the work of both ministers and physicians in the seventeenth and eighteenth centuries must not be forgotten as we seek to interpret their writings. Against this backcloth we can see that preindustrial Puritan preachers likely felt little need to explicitly justify the then patently obvious claim that many diseases were in fact the wages of sin—particularly those that resulted from a manifest disregard for God's law. This fact of life was not, as Warner might claim, empirically self-evident and immune to culturally informed presuppositions. It was instead itself a well-established cultural inheritance widely shared by seventeenth- and eighteenth-century Protestants. For those ensconced in this common culture, symptoms of culpable diseases may not themselves have exhibited "choices," the free will of the afflicted, but they nonetheless quite certainly bore the stigma of sin and God's disfavor.

Diseases such as leprosy and the pox were widely thought to follow from sinful sexual behavior, dropsy and madness from gluttony, and so on (Thomas 1971). For many early modern Protestants these were very real diseases, but diseases that invited contempt rather than sympathy. They were diseases that marked one as an unregenerate sinner, damned and deserving not of care but of all the brutality one could anticipate from hell. As Richard Baxter ([1673] 1825, 410–11) advised, "Involuntary madness deserveth compassion, but voluntary madness, the sharpest whips." Hence, the questions that have hitherto framed much of the debate on the medicalization of addiction—when, where, and how addiction was transformed from a sin into a sickness—don't fully square with the historical record. We should instead be asking when, where, and how the sinful sickness of habitual drunkenness became a cause for compassion rather than contempt. What changed was not the status of habitual drunkenness as a sinful sickness but the status of those perceived to be afflicted from damned and despised to reformable and deserving of support. Before the middle of the eighteenth century, habitual drunkards were often described as pathologically enslaved to drink or drunkenness (Nicholls 2009; Porter 1985; Warner 1994). What was largely missing was any expression of empathy for those so enslaved or any faith that they could or should be freed from their madness.

The early modern Puritan discourse on freedom and addiction was predicated on the doctrine of predestination, a doctrine that strictly opposed the idea that our eternal fate was a reward of virtue or punishment of vice. Vicious and virtuous conduct were held to issue not from a provisional character capable of moral corruption or elevation but instead from a fixed and eternal character either damned or saved from the outset. Freedom, as opposed to the slavery of habitual drunkenness, was understood as the conduct of one's life in accordance with the dictates of a morally ordered universe. It reflected one's status among the elect and the happy harmony of one's own rational judgment with God's will. Conversely, the sin of habitual drunkenness was understood as a form of slavery to Satan rather than, as liberal theorists would have it today, an independently chosen moral transgression.[5] One was punished as a minion of Satan rather than, as now, an autonomous and reformable wrongdoer. It was within this discursive frame that the logic of brutally forsaking those enslaved by alcohol made moral sense.

The early modern rise of civic republicanism rather dramatically reoriented thinking on these matters (Nicholls 2009; Schmidt 1995). In contrast to Puritan thought, this orientation to freedom was predicated not on abstract scholastic dialogue regarding the fixed characteristics of the immaterial human soul and its worldly tribulations but on mundane practical dialogue through which was fluidly shaped one's eminently cultivated and worldly personal character. Civic republican conceptions of freedom and slavery can be traced back to ancient Greek and Roman political thought, but, via the Italian renaissance, they enjoyed a notable comeback in seventeenth-century England (Pocock 1975). For civic republicans, freedom consisted in our use of reason both to tame our unruly and selfish passions and to develop and implement an educated understanding of the public good. This was in its orthodox form a plainly aristocratic ethos whereby men of excellence exhibited their distinction through wise and honorable public service.

However, its revival in early modern England reflected a much more dynamic public culture contested by royal, aristocratic, religious, and commercial actors, among others (Withington 2007). This social structural context had the effect of shifting early modern orientations to reason and freedom from state-centric aristocratic virtues such as courage and honor in the direction of more civic virtues such as mundane sensibility, tact, and diplomacy (Knott 2009; Wood 1998, x). Slavery consisted in one's capacity to realize these virtues being denied through unreasoned servitude (Pocock 1975, 229).

Crucially for present purposes, the capacity to develop these virtues could be denied not only by the tyranny of others but also by the tyranny of our own passions and desires. By civic republican lights, slavery to habitual drunkenness was less an exhibit of one's fixed status among the damned than a profligate but acquired propensity to debase one's character—an unchecked desire for excessive (and therefore "unnatural") bodily enjoyment eclipsing one's commitment to act and reason soundly for the public good. Moreover, yielding to temptation was understood not as a mark of one's fixed status as eternally damned but as a disabling *process* whereby one became progressively more dissipated, enervated, and enslaved the more one continued to yield (Berry 1994).

During the eighteenth century, one could increasingly observe invocations of civic republican themes among those concerned that the luxury and license of the prosperous were pervading society to an extent that threatened the nation's survival (Reith 2019). For example, in his highly influential tract *An Enquiry into the Causes of the Late Increase in Robbers*, Henry Fielding (1751, 6) writes,

> First then, I think, that the vast Torrent of Luxury which of late Years hath poured itself into this Nation, hath greatly contributed to produce, among many others, the Mischief I here complain of. I am not here to satirize the Great, among whom Luxury is probably rather a moral than a political Evil. But Vices no more than Diseases will stop with them; for bad Habits are as infectious by Example, as the Plague itself by Contact. In free Countries, at least, it is a Branch of Liberty claimed by the People to be as wicked and as profligate as their Superiors.

Though his primary concern was the corrupting effects of the spread of luxury and license to the lower orders of society, Fielding (1751, 6) made plain his view that these effects were evident throughout all the strata of English society and that they hailed in the first instance from the highest strata. This spread of profligacy was exacerbated by the growth in trade and the material prosperity that came with it (Fielding 1751, xxiv). Wealth was distracting the English people from virtue and thereby from both true freedom and good health. As Fielding's writing illustrates, civic republican arguments provided a timely opportunity for Protestant reformers and others to join forces in opposition to both the lusty indulgences of the crown and court and those of the increasingly ubiquitous men of commerce. It was they who were to blame for enticing the morally and intellectually vulnerable working classes into extravagant and unnatural habits that, while immoral among the better sort, were positively ruinous for the poor, particularly poor women and children. This trend was not only enervating and enslaving individuals but the nation as a whole by making the "useful" ranks of the population morally, intellectually, and physically unfit. Few of the corrupting effects of luxury received more attention than the abuse of distilled spirits.

By the time Benjamin Rush and Thomas Trotter, widely regarded as the fathers of addiction medicine, lent their authority to the notion that habitual drunkenness is a genuine disease, the general contours of their arguments had become all but commonplace among civic republican patriots (Nicholls 2009). These arguments were dedicated to stemming the rot of royal and aristocratic indulgence and caprice, the amoral and licentious pursuit of profit through trade, and the growing depravity and disorder they observed in the increasingly overflowing and overwhelmed urban centers. Translating republican concerns for the vicious temptations of luxury and license into the quasi-medical language of nervous overstimulation, natural and unnatural passions, the arguments of Rush and Trotter reiterated broader anxieties regarding the political, social, moral, and medical dangers of overindulgence and, in particular, the growing temptations in this regard introduced by growing wealth, modern civilization, and urban life (Porter 1992). And like their civic republican compatriots, Rush and Trotter located the cure for addiction in the embrace of temperance, personal bonds, modest living, and the refuge of the agrarian countryside. Freedom from addiction, then, both could and should be fostered through the moderation of nervous stimulation and the suppression of desires to satiate the unnatural passions provoked and unleashed by the dazzle of urban life.

While thinkers like Trotter and Rush were plainly concerned about the dark side of their growing consumer societies and the proliferating and increasingly potent temptations to which people were ever more routinely exposed, they were not wholly critical or pessimistic regarding modernization. Rush, in particular, was in much of his writing quite hopeful that postrevolutionary America would become a bastion of republican egalitarianism from which the rest of the world might draw inspiration. Unprecedented religious and political freedoms would enrich and empower the United States while also rendering them havens of Christian and republican virtue (D'Elia 1974). While some people might require tutelage and encouragement to meet their civic republican obligations, he did not for a moment see this as incompatible with the flourishing of religious, political, and cultural freedoms he believed were the hallmarks of his young nation. For Rush, the promotion of republican virtues was entirely compatible with free inquiry, candor, and a robust tolerance of difference and dissent. Pace predestinarian Puritans, then, he believed recovery from addiction was eminently achievable through temperance. And temperance was emphatically not a matter of slavish devotion to received medical, moral, or political doctrine but of inclusive, sociable, and self-critical dialogue and debate.

Concluding Remarks

In early modern Puritan distinctions between living in conformity or opposition to the divine dictates of nature and in civic republican distinctions between natural and unnatural passions, one can rather easily discern genealogical precursors to the distinction NIDA brain disease boosters now draw between natural and unnatural rewards. However, unlike today's neurologists, early modern commentators had the discursive advantage of grounding their distinctions in a Lockean natural universe as yet still saturated in largely Protestant moral meaning, a natural universe putatively designed providentially with direct respect to humanity's moral freedom, to encourage virtue and good health and to discourage vice and physical enervation. Pressed by contemporary scientific standards to conceive of human nature in universal and value-neutral terms as a wholly biomechanical product of natural selection, brain disease theorists are now left largely bereft of conceptual resources with which to link their biologically deterministic accounts of health and illness to the vicissitudes of virtue and freedom. As we have seen, the effective conflation of freedom with the narrow pursuit of health and reproduction through natural rewards simply doesn't hold up against the more liberal conceptions of freedom that have come to dominate both our contemporary scientific and popular cultural imaginations.

Conversely, though, the presumptively universal and value-neutral liberal ontology of freedom one finds in much addiction science leaves us largely bereft of conceptual resources with which to account for the experiences of attenuated freedom; alienation from our thoughts, feelings, and behavior; or any manner of genuine *mental* affliction (and hence any convincing intellectual warrant for compassion rather than contempt for putative addicts). Instead, it is widely held as axiomatic that all preferences exhibited by a particular person are also the preferences of that person's self.[6] However, as an empirical matter, we must acknowledge that people do occasionally exhibit behavior radically inconsistent with the ordinary proclivities they and others normally find characteristic of their particular selves and that such inconsistencies often serve both in clinical settings and in everyday life as empirical grounds for relinquishing the faith that they have freely or deliberately chosen to so behave and, indeed, as warrants for therapeutic care (Weinberg 2005).

A review of the early modern discursive registers considered here highlights first of all that when it comes to understanding the relationship between freedom and addiction, history does in fact furnish alternatives to the now widely reified antinomy between ontological liberalism and biological determinism. Indeed, I would argue that the more fluid and dynamic dichotomy between freedom and slavery that preoccupied early modern thinkers is a far more apt one for understanding addiction than is the much more rigid contemporary dichotomy between freedom and biological determinism. Second, a consideration of these discursive registers also highlights the considerable intersection that was once taken for granted between judgments of freedom and judgments of virtue and vice. Whereas we now tend to see virtuous and vicious conduct as equally free, early modern thinkers were much more inclined to see vicious conduct to exhibit some manner of slavery to Satan, one's baser passions, or both. Perhaps our understanding of the contemporary lived experience of addiction and its relation to freedom would be well served by a reconsideration of the extent to which addicts and/or their significant others might be somehow similarly predisposed and indeed what, if any, revisions to the liberal regard for freedom and addiction this might suggest.

As is well known, modern liberalism owes much to the legacy of the Scottish Enlightenment. In the eighteenth century, Francis Hutcheson insisted that humans are endowed with a moral sense that provides for our learning from, and correcting, our moral errors. David Hume added that it is through the experience of pain in the face of vice and pleasure in the face of virtue that this moral sense is psychologically realized. By way of Adam Smith and, later, utilitarians such as Jeremy Bentham and John Stuart Mill, this naturalized and sentimentalized conception of good and evil was fused with a broader conception of personal preference and transformed into a general conception of human rationality predicated on the pursuit of happiness (D. Levine 1995). Confluent as it was with sociohistorical trends toward religious and ethical pluralism, parliamentary democracy, and free-market capitalism, the utilitarian conception of the self as autonomous happiness maximizer has become far and away the most influential of the modern era and remains fundamental to the liberal creed.

But, by these lights, there can be no distinction between what we desire and what we consider good because our only measure of goodness is what we desire. As we have seen, this makes distinguishing freedom from the pursuit of what we desire axiomatically impossible and, hence, conceptualizing the idea of enslavement to one's desires—that is, addiction—equally impossible. Moreover, individuals cannot be mistaken in this regard because for anyone to take issue with the individual's desires is, by definition, an act of oppressive interference with their free and autonomous pursuit of happiness. But this rigid orthodoxy of extreme moral agnosticism is plainly inconsistent with how people, as an empirical matter, normally orient to their own and one another's conduct in their everyday lives. In practice, we routinely evaluate whether our own and one another's desires are or are not good for us or for those around us. And these moral evaluations are contingent on a vast range of contextual considerations (Weinberg 2005; Zigon 2011). Hence, if we are to reconcile liberal theory to the manifest empirical contingency of judgments concerning freedom and addiction, it will be immensely helpful, drawing our cues from early modern thought, to distinguish between contemporary liberal theory's preponderantly hedonic orientation to personal values and what Aristotle called eudaemonic values.[7]

Unlike hedonic values, eudaemonic values are not constituted by individual desires alone. Indeed, they are values that may very well clash with our desires and with which our behavior may, even chronically, fail to conform. This allows for a liberal, or individualized and multicultural, appreciation for the broad range of values that may orient free and autonomous behavior without thereby assuming these values are invariably hedonic. It thereby creates a possibility for conceptualizing disjuncture and tension between our desires and our free agency and hence our addictions, without capitulating to the fraught conceptual antinomy between freedom and biological determinism. Liberal critics of the brain disease paradigm are no doubt correct to note the empirically untenable narrowness of the neurological equation of freedom with the rational pursuit of natural rewards. But, contrary to these liberal critics, perhaps it is more empirically tenable, therapeutically useful, and humane to view the experience of freedom among those who consider themselves addicts as embodied in the work they do themselves and in collaboration with others to live more consistently in line with the eudaemonic values they consider conducive to their personal and social flourishing rather than continuing to adhere to the widely, if not uniformly, held liberal ontological doctrine that freedom is only ever to be found in the pursuit of pleasure.

Returning, then, to the contemporary project of providing scientific warrant for therapeutic care over blame and punishment, we might observe that sometimes, and for a variety of biological, psychological, and social reasons, we may become sufficiently alienated from certain of our habitual desires that we cease to experience them as genuinely our own and instead feel them as afflictions and in some sense enslaving. Whereas much of contemporary addiction science now assumes a more or less unified human subject possessed of habits largely integrated through cost-benefit analysis, research in neurology, psychology, and sociology is beginning to more fully appreciate the reality of subjective fragmentation and disunity. For example, the distinguished neurologist of addiction and critic of the brain disease discourse Marc Lewis has written in this regard that habit learning originates piecemeal in setting specific kinds of ways but that eventually, because brains tend to conserve structure and resources, habits, or acquired "synaptic networks," often converge and become mutually reinforcing. However, he notes, these processes need not converge on a wholly unified subject, or fully integrated hub, for all experience, deliberation, and volition. Instead, "alternative synaptic networks can compete with each other. . . . This is the case when addiction arises in development, but also when it dissipates, replaced by the desire for and belief in alternative outcomes" (M. Lewis 2017b, 182).

What Lewis doesn't specify, however, and what prevents him from reconciling his incisive understanding of the neurology of addiction with his hope to produce a warrant for therapeutic care, is the labile and dynamic relationships that occur between the diverse constellations of habitual desire he describes as the neuroplastic synaptic networks to be found in our biomechanical brains, on the one hand, and, on the other hand, our *selves* specifically as self-controlling, self-discovering, self-actualizing, and ethically accountable. The fact that such selves can be, and indeed too often actually are, genuinely alienated from and afflicted by deeply habituated desires perceived and often dreaded as traumatizing, dangerous, or, at the very least, profoundly ethically inconsistent with who they are or wish to be provides robust warrant for therapeutic care. And it is precisely the emancipation and empowerment of these selves over their addictions that therapeutic care for addicts often is, and ought to be, designed to foster.

LINDESMITH ON ADDICTION
A Critical History of a Classic Theory

Alfred Lindesmith was not the first sociologist to give sustained consideration to deviant drug use (Brown 193 I; Dai 1937); however, he was the first sociologist to develop a distinctively sociological approach to the phenomenon. Lindesmith's most influential research focused on the nature of heroin addiction and is still considered by many the classic sociological theory of addiction (Akers 1992; McAuliffe and Gordon 1974; Stephens 1991). His theoretical achievement was to show that in addition to affecting the body biochemically, drugs, and the experiences their ingestion produces, are meaningful to people in ways that cannot be reduced to the interactions of a chemical agent with a human physiological system.

Nevertheless, Lindesmith's manner of conceptually distinguishing between meaningful experiences and physiological processes has had important limiting effects on sociological research. According to his account, opiates biochemically alter objective physiological states within the body. These biochemical changes are said to cause brute *physical* sensations that arise as meaningful contents of human consciousness only to the extent they have been *mindfully* subjected to symbolically mediated interpretation (Lindesmith 1938a, 1938b, 1947, 1965b, 1968). Because Lindesmith construed meaningful experience exclusively in terms of symbolically mediated perception, he was forced to posit a strict dualism between *cognitively* apprehended perceptual events (which were, by definition, symbolically mediated and therefore socially learned and socially constituted) and *physically* apprehended perceptual events (which were, by definition, unmediated brute sensations caused solely by physical stimuli and therefore impervious to social influences). This mind-body dualism is untenable on both epistemological and phenomenological grounds (Leder 1990) and inhibits conceptually rigorous sociological contributions to our understanding of the visceral, or prereflective and nonsymbolic, features of drug use and drug-induced experience.

In this chapter, I provide a critical history of the evolution of Lindesmith's theory of addiction in an effort to demonstrate the intellectual currents and controversies in which, and for which, it took form. I thus endeavor not only to point out its strengths and weaknesses in light of contemporary sociological concerns but also to make historical sense of the successive developments of his theory in light of the specific debates that gave rise to them. I conclude by outlining a praxiological alternative to Lindesmith's semiotic approach to the meaningful experience of drug effects. The proposed alternative draws upon the work of contemporary social theorists who have attended to the ways in which we are transformed through praxis at a prereflective, nonsymbolic level of being (Bourdieu 1990; Coulter 1994; Merleau-Ponty 1962; Ostrow 1990; Shusterman 1991). This praxiological rubric both preserves the epistemological gains Lindesmith made in his emphasis on meaning as a crucial component in the addiction process and overcomes the limitations of his mind-body dualism.

Lindesmith the Psychical Interactionist

Alfred Lindesmith first formulated his theory of addiction in the 1930s, as a graduate student of Herbert Blumer at the University of Chicago (Lindesmith 1938b, 593). At that time, the sociology department at Chicago was fiercely divided between the followers and allies of William Fielding Ogburn, a positivist statistician, and the antipositivist followers of the so-called psychical interactionist school, which included W. I. Thomas, Charles Horton Cooley, and Herbert Blumer (Bannister 1987; Hammersley 1989). Blumer, in particular, was a vocal defender of psychical interactionism and qualitative sociological research methods against the determinism, positivism, and quantitative methods that he felt were beginning to dominate the discipline of sociology (Blumer 1931). Drawing on the work of another University of Chicago scholar, George Herbert Mead, Blumer (1937, 1969) vigorously critiqued quantitative sociology and advocated what he regarded as the more theoretically sophisticated and naturalistic style of sociology he came to call "symbolic interactionism."

Lindesmith took after his mentor in a number of important respects. His theory of drug addiction was based on unstructured interviews with approximately fifty heroin addicts and was explicitly cast as a theoretical and methodological exemplar for rigorous qualitative social science (Lindesmith 1938b, 609). And, like his mentor, Lindesmith made the symbolically mediated interpretations his subjects conferred on their actions and experiences the central element of his theory.

In order to properly place Lindesmith's theory in its historical and intellectual context, however, we must also look beyond the peculiarities of the scientific field within sociology to the place of sociology as a whole in the larger scientific field of American academia during this period.[1] A sociological theory of addiction was not only of interest to sociologists but was also in competition with medical, psychiatric, and psychological theories of addiction. Indeed, Lindesmith's (1938b) article provoked immediate opposition from Dr. David Slight, a psychiatrist at the University of Chicago, whose comment (Slight 1938) appeared in the same issue of the *American Journal of Sociology* as did the original article and Lindesmith's (1938a) rejoinder.

Lindesmith's reply to Slight presaged his extensive writings in criticism of medical and psychoanalytic theories, which he felt did not sufficiently attend to the "cognitive factors" that accompany the development of addiction (Lindesmith 1940b, 1965b, 1968). He criticized medical and psychoanalytic theories for defining addicts post hoc as people seeking in drugs an escape from their intrinsic personal defects. It is plainly nonsociological to explain addiction with respect to intrinsic personal pathologies, and Lindesmith argued persuasively that theories that did so were not sufficient as general theories of the phenomenon. As he rightly pointed out, they could not account for the circumstances under which personal pathology would or would not cause addiction to occur, nor the large number of people who were to all appearances quite normal before their addictions had ensued.

Instead of looking for predisposing factors or the generic characteristics of an "addictive personality," Lindesmith emphasized the *process* of becoming addicted and argued that the symbolic meanings drug users communicated to one another regarding the effects of opiates was essential to the transformation of a nonaddicted heroin user into a heroin addict. Focusing on the symbolic categories drug users ostensibly applied in their interpretations of drug effects and positing them as essential to the production of addiction, he highlighted language and interaction—two phenomena that were squarely sociological.

The sociologist Charles Camic (1986) has shown the extent to which American sociologists in the first half of the twentieth century were concerned to distinguish and defend their conceptual repertoire against the encroachment of more powerful academic disciplines, particularly psychology. He makes his case specifically with respect to the concept of habit. Camic shows that while noted masters of sociological theory, such as Émile Durkheim and Max Weber, conferred considerable sociological importance on the notion of habit, American sociologists in the early twentieth century elided the topic from their own concerns due to pressures exerted from outside sociology: "This dramatic change [was] a result of the interdisciplinary disputes that surrounded the institutionalization of sociology as an academic discipline, particularly sociology's struggles with behaviorist psychology, which had by then projected into prominence a notion of habit deriving from 19th century biological thought" (Camic 1986, 1039–40).

Camic argues that American sociologists grew disenchanted with the notion of habit primarily due to the firm hold on the concept by Watsonian behaviorists in psychology who threatened to abrogate sociology's precarious footing in the academy. Nowhere was this aversive reaction stronger than among the psychical interactionists at the University of Chicago. W. I. Thomas, who earlier in his career had embraced the concept of habit, came to denounce its limits in specifically sociological research.

> Thomas unequivocally reversed his once-positive stance toward physiology and likewise toward habit. Now, deeming unacceptable ". . . the principles recently developed by the behavioristic school," particularly its "indistinct [application] of the term 'habit' to [all] uniformities of behavior," he bluntly declared that "'habit' . . . should be restricted to the biological field; [for it] involves no conscious, purposeful regulation of [conduct], but merely . . . is unreflective. . . . The uniformity of behavior [that constitutes social life] is not a uniformity of organic habits but of consciously followed rules." (Camic 1986, 1072)

Without the conceptual resources at hand to navigate between the Scylla of "conscious, purposeful regulation of [conduct]" and the Charybdis of Watsonian behaviorism, Thomas opted for the former. He thereby ushered in an era in American sociology that has been widely characterized by a rigid analytic dualism between cognitive and bodily processes wherein the scope of reflective consciousness in human agency has been profoundly overemphasized (Bourdieu 1990; Camic 1986; Ostrow 1990). Lindesmith's (1938b, 597–98) sociological theory of addiction bears the marks of this general theoretical trend: "In this paper the term 'habituated' will be used to refer to the development of the mere physiological tolerance, whereas the term 'addiction' will be reserved for application to cases in which there is added to the physiological or pharmacological tolerance a psychic addiction which is marked by the appearance of an imperious desire for the drug."

Here, Lindesmith distinguishes "desire" as a psychic phenomenon from "mere physiological tolerance," which, while it may speak to the brute bodily processes underlying addiction, does not explain the subjective experience for which he reserves the term *addiction*. Accordingly, addicts must reflect on the source of their physiological symptoms for the behavior characteristic of addiction to arise (Lindesmith 1938b, 606). In Lindesmith's view, certain physical sensations occurred as unmediated outcomes of the objective biochemical changes introduced by the administration of opiates to the human nervous system. But he construed the *meaning* and *practical relevance* of these brute physical sensations exclusively in terms of conscious awareness mediated by the "significant symbols" provided by society (Lindesmith 1938b, 606–7). Thus the meaning, and indeed every learned aspect, of drug-induced behavior and experience was viewed as occurring exclusively through symbolically mediated *mental* processes, in contrast to drug-induced *physical* sensations, which were considered brute experiences that did not implicate meaning, learning, social life, or practical action.

According to Lindesmith's earliest statements, it was the mental apprehension of physical sensations—that is, the consciously attended and symbolically mediated meaning that drug-induced physical sensations had for people—that determined whether or not they became addicts. Lindesmith's statement of his theory in his first book, *Opiate Addiction* (1947), also remains completely consonant with the psychical interactionists' cognitivist strategies of theoretical resistance to Watsonian behaviorism. Reiterating his emphasis on conscious reflection and the symbolically mediated meaning of drug effects, Lindesmith continued to argue for two necessary and sufficient conditions for the emergence of addiction: first, the occurrence of physiological symptoms of withdrawal from the drug; and second, their conscious interpretation as such (as mediated through language) and the consumption of the drug for the conscious purpose of alleviating withdrawal symptoms. Through at least 1947, Lindesmith (1947, 46) remained emphatic in his insistence on the conscious and reflective character of addictive craving: "That addiction is characterized by intense desire for the drug scarcely needs elaboration; however, it should be emphasized that this craving is self-conscious and its object is known."

Lindesmith and Behaviorism

Lindesmith's concern to underscore the conscious quality of the addict's craving for opiates begins to wane, however, beginning with his 1965 essay "Problems in the Social Psychology of Addiction." Here, he begins to adopt some of the conceptual language of behavioral psychology—a theoretical rubric noted for its studious avoidance of any references to such "inner" processes as thought, meaning, interpretation, or consciousness—to express his theoretical position.

> The addict's craving . . . is not a rational assessment or choice of any sort, but basically an irrational compulsion arising from the repetition of a sequence of experiences in a process like that which leads to a conditioned response. It is assumed that the principal difference between the consequences of the conditioning process in human beings and lower animals lies in the fact that human beings are capable of conceptual thought and language behavior, and therefore the craving is symbolically elaborated, and responses arising from it are directed or controlled by conceptual processes. (Lindesmith 1965b, 136)

Even if we ignore the conceptual tension inherent in Lindesmith's apparent effort to fuse Blumer's voluntarist and cognitivist understanding of meaning and social learning with the behaviorists' determinist and emphatically antimentalist notion of conditioned reflexes, the language of this paragraph is still puzzling. Why at this late date in his career did Lindesmith begin using the language of conditioning, a language traditionally so subversive to his own scientific predilections?

Two explanations seem possible. One suggests that Lindesmith was simply responding to new research. In 1965, behavioral psychologist John Nichols (1965) published the results of research in which he had achieved relapsing behavior in rats. This could not have been anticipated by Lindesmith's theory because rats lack the linguistic skills he had insisted were necessary prerequisites to one of his essential features of the addiction process—the symbolic interpretation of withdrawal symptoms specifically as withdrawal symptoms. Prior to this work, Lindesmith (1947, 168–70) had repeatedly held that in the absence of linguistic competence, neither addiction nor relapsing behavior could occur.

However, in *Addiction and Opiates,* the substantially revised version of his first book, Lindesmith (1968, 126–27) added a detailed discussion of Nichols's work and confessed that he was incorrect in his original belief that "relapse behavior had never been induced in lower animals and probably could not be." It might be argued that Lindesmith was simply persuaded that learning processes that are not symbolically mediated are important determinants of addiction and relapse and he had therefore integrated references to them into his own work. However, one point militates strongly against such a conclusion. Despite his concession regarding relapse in rats and his adoption of the language of conditioning, Lindesmith remained extremely resistant to the notion that "lower animals" can become addicts in the same sense as can human beings. His statements with respect to the animal studies, and the behaviorist orientation to addiction they seemed to support, are in large part a defense of the essential role of language and thought in the addiction process. Thus Lindesmith (1968, 194) still insisted that "children and animals cannot become addicts because they lack the ability to use and respond to the complex linguistic structures which have grown up in human society."

Why, then, did he adopt the language of conditioning if he was not prepared to capitulate to behaviorism? The most plausible explanation is that his well-known commitment to a therapeutic societal response to the addict demanded that he do so. Lindesmith was not merely an academic social theorist; indeed, he wrote of the dangers inherent in assuming theoretical postures that are not sensitive to the realities of policy reform (Lindesmith 1960). His tireless advocacy for decriminalizing addiction and providing addicts with medical treatment has been well documented (Conrad and Schneider 1992, 130). However, if we look closely at the theoretical implications of the Blumerian social psychology Lindesmith adopted in his early work, we discover it is not capable of sustaining his policy position.

Blumer's (1969) theoretical emphasis of meaning, interpretation, the self, and the importance of self-indication in human agency embodied a conscious effort to resist both psychologically and social structurally deterministic visions of the social act. Rather than being *acted on* by objective social and psychological structures, human agents were conceptualized as symbolically imbuing the world with meaning in order to facilitate their own chosen projects (Blumer 1969, 78–89). By conceptually distinguishing between the structures of the objective world and their symbolic interpretation by human agents, Blumer insisted on a voluntaristic understanding of social action that highlighted people's freedom from both social and psychological determinism (Lewis and Smith 1980). In this way he defended naturalistic and qualitative studies of social life against those structural determinists (be they sociological, psychological, or biological) who would disparage the rigor and the relevance of such studies.

Obviously, then, Blumer's social psychology could not and was specifically not intended to explain the learning processes through which people might develop a sense that their perceptions and actions *were* beyond their willful capacity to control and hence that they were determined by social, psychological, or biological structures. Blumer's social psychology was therefore incapable of showing how drug addiction could be suffered rather than chosen, and it offered no theoretical rationale for Lindesmith's demand that society respond to addiction with medical treatment rather than criminal punishment. Blumer himself recognized this when he excluded drug craving from his field of analysis:

> I submit that a realistic analysis of the human act shows that the tendency to act cannot be taken as moulding or controlling the act. At best the tendency or preparation to act is merely an element that enters into the developing act—no more than an initial bid for a possible line of action. There are, of course, the relatively infrequent cases wherein the tendency seems to dominate the act to the exclusion of the demands of the situation and the expectations of others—cases such as mood of melancholy, *the cravings of a drug addict for narcotics,* a burning rage, and fright in a panic. *These are instances in which there is no process of self-indication,* or, as we commonly say, instances in which the individual "loses his head." (Blumer 1969, 97, emphasis added)

Lindesmith (1965b, 136) also recognized the problem, and, without theoretically justifying or explicitly working through the tenability of his position, drew upon the language of conditioning only to insist that "the addict's craving . . . is not a rational assessment or choice of any sort, but basically an irrational compulsion." The difficulty is that he did not tell us how we might theoretically reconcile addicts' putative "irrational compulsion" to interpret and respond to given physical sensations specifically as irresistible cravings for narcotics with Blumer's antideterministic view of meaningful experience and social learning. Nor did he seem to repudiate the Blumerian approach to meaning and social learning. We are thus left to speculate as to the mechanism(s) by which a pattern of practical action and interpretation learned according to the principles of Blumer's voluntaristic social psychology could ever assume the compulsively *involuntary* character that Lindesmith suggests characterizes the opiate addict's craving for and use of narcotics. Given the strict mind-body dualism inherent in the Blumerian approach to meaning and social learning, it is extremely difficult to envision how any learned pattern of interpretation and/or practical action could come to be suffused with the level of emotional urgency and irrepressibility that Lindesmith insisted was the hallmark of craving and addictive behavior.

Insofar as he did not resolve this issue, Lindesmith did not adequately provide for the analytic possibility of a learning process through which addicts might progressively *lose* control over their actions and interpretations. Nor was he any longer justified, following the animal studies, in insisting that "the ability to use and respond to complex linguistic structures" is an essential prerequisite to the addiction process (Lindesmith 1968, 194). The animal studies showed that linguistic skills are not necessary for the occurrence of learning processes through which prolonged self-destructive attachments to the use of drugs take place. Lindesmith's statements that these attachments do not amount to addiction are based on, rather than empirically supportive of, the principle that only linguistically competent adult human beings can become addicts and a wider faith in the centrality of language and symbolic mediation to all meaningful human action. His later statements thus ceased to "provide a place for the exceptional or crucial case" (Lindesmith 1938b, 609) and became instead a problematic effort to extend a particular scientific ideology regarding distinctively human conduct.

Moving beyond Lindesmith's Mind-Body Dualism

I have argued that the trajectory in which Lindesmith's theory of addiction evolved can best be understood as a product of historically specific academic and political conflicts that pitted qualitative sociologists against quantitative sociologists; the fledgling discipline of sociology against medicine, psychiatry, and psychology; and advocates of therapy for addicts against those who would simply punish them. By successfully promoting the view that meaning and social learning are essential components of the addiction process, Lindesmith secured a jurisdiction for qualitative sociology in drug studies. Unfortunately, he was not able to reconcile his manner of theoretically emphasizing meaning and social learning with his campaign to decriminalize and medicalize addiction.

Thus, while as sociologists we might justifiably wish to thank Alfred Lindesmith for his successful advocacy of our discipline and for more hu-

mane societal responses to addicts, we must acknowledge that modern sociological theorizing is, nonetheless, encumbered by his legacy. New scientific
challenges are upon us and we must ensure that our theoretical resources are
adequate to our current research needs. Fundamental to this project must be
a reconceptualization of the phenomenology of drug-induced behavior and
experience. We must move beyond the mind-body dualism inherent in the
Blumerian social psychology that has hitherto informed our work.

Following Lindesmith, sociological parlance has remained largely loyal to
the view that the meaningful experience and practical relevance of drug effects are constituted in symbolically mediated interpretations of the brute
physical sensations produced by psychoactive drugs (H. Becker 1953, 1967;
Biernacki 1986; Denzin 1993; Stephens 1991). This position has served to
highlight the importance of sociological research on drug problems by under-
scoring the centrality of meaning and social learning to the lived experience
of drug effects. However, construing meaning in exclusively symbolic terms
inhibits the production of conceptually rigorous sociological contributions
to our understanding of the nonsymbolic features of human drug use and
drug-induced experience.

Sociologists have often assumed that the visceral features of drug effects
are properly construed as brute physical sensations produced solely by the
presence of psychoactive drugs in the body. They have thus conceptualized
these features as distinct from, and experientially prior to, the methods that
drug users learn for meaningfully appreciating them. While this approach
may account for some of the gross physiological reactions to certain drugs, it
fails to provide for analyses of the sociogenic influences that have an impact
on the character of visceral drug effects or the widely noted variations in visceral effect that a given drug may produce across different practical settings.
For example, it cannot explain Norman Zinberg's (1984) finding that alcohol
may act as a relaxant under one set of circumstances and a stimulant under
another. Furthermore, it can tell us nothing about the visceral compulsions
to use drugs that some people experience even when drugs are *not* present in
their bodies. Lindesmith (1968, 154) sought to account for such drug-related,
but not drug-induced, visceral experiences among former heroin addicts by
suggesting they were subconscious generalizations to other forms of stress
of addicts' interpretive and behavioral response to withdrawal distress. If it
were to be made clear how visceral sensations might drive symbolic interpretations under Lindesmith's Blumerian social psychology, this explanation
might account for some of the cravings people feel for drugs that do indeed
produce physiological withdrawal symptoms. But it does not explain cravings

for drugs such as nicotine and crack cocaine, which do not produce gross physiological withdrawal symptoms (Gawin 1991). Nor does it jibe well with the recurrent finding that former heroin addicts do not necessarily experience craving indiscriminately in response to any extrinsic source of stress. Contra Lindesmith, many addicts become stressed only after they begin craving drugs in response to circumstances deemed similar to those in which they had formerly used (Robins 1993; Waldorf 1983).

These limitations of, and anomalies for, received sociological theory can be overcome if we forgo the analytic dualism between mental and physical perception implicit in Blumerian social psychology. Epistemologists and phenomenologists have offered a litany of arguments that proclaim the analytic untenability of the notion that human perception can be divided into the body's passive apprehension of unmediated brute physical sensations and the mind's active symbolic interpretation of their meaning (Dreyfus 1991; Leder 1990; Merleau-Ponty 1962; Polanyi 1962; Rorty 1979; Shusterman 1991; Taylor 1993; Wittgenstein 1958). If we heed these arguments and join the growing number of social theorists who have come to recognize that meaningful experience often takes place at a prereflective, nonsymbolic, visceral level of being (Bourdieu 1990; Calhoun 1995; Coulter and Parsons 1990; Ostrow 1990), the theoretical problems discussed here can be resolved.

By the lights of a *praxiological* approach to meaning and social learning, the meanings and practical relevances that attach to drugs and to the effects of their ingestion should not be understood as acquired exclusively through processes of *learning to symbolically represent* drug-induced experiences but also through processes of *learning to use* drugs as resources in given fields of practical action. It is not necessary that people linguistically categorize drugs and/or engage in some manner of dialogue regarding their effects in order to develop subtle competencies regarding the perception and operationalization of those effects in practical action. Indeed, animals that apparently lack language skills altogether are capable of such learning, and so language cannot be posited as an essential feature of it. It is only necessary that people become convinced there are uses to which they can put given drugs and come to incorporate drug use into the conduct of their lives. Through such learning processes, people will develop what Bourdieu (1990) has called a "practical sense" for the uses of drugs quite apart from their capacities to symbolically represent those uses.

This approach suggests that if under particular practical conditions drug use is experienced as conducive to competent performance, it will quite likely become incorporated into a person's repertoire of techniques for coping with similar practical conditions. Again, this acquired repertoire of coping techniques must be understood in fundamentally praxiological terms. It is not a stored system of symbolic knowledge, nor a set of techniques for merely interpreting (or representing) given settings. Rather, it is more properly understood as a presymbolic set of embodied dispositions, or *habitus,* that acts as a loosely organized but largely setting-specific "schemata of perception and appreciation" (Bourdieu and Wacquant 1992, 14). This habitus is acquired in and for actively responding to the perceived demands of particular practical environments.[2]

For example, people may find themselves viscerally drawn to the use of alcohol in order to relax after a long day at work or to stimulate their playful participation in the goings-on of a party, if indeed they have found the use of alcohol conducive to the accomplishment of such projects in the past. The visceral experiences that follow from, as well as those that incline one toward, the use of a drug can thus be understood as deriving in some significant part from the historically and culturally specific contexts in which and for which one has tacitly learned to use the drug. Obviously, if use of the drug has not been experienced as conducive to meeting the demands of a given practical environment, it will be unlikely to inspire future craving or visceral inclination toward its use in homologous environments.

Drug problems arise when people, or their significant others, perceive that their tacit reliance on a drug for coping in one area of their lives has a negative impact on their coping in that or other areas. According to the phenomenology I am proposing here, this perception is often not enough to produce cessation of drug use because the inclination to use does not manifest in lived experience as a deliberate decision, let alone a holistic cost-benefit analysis, but as a visceral impulse informed by the perceived practical demands of the moment. The inclination to use drugs is thus experienced as deriving from beyond the self and decidedly not in any way a deliberate exercise of self-will.[3] However, the difficulties thus experienced may occur with various degrees of intensity depending on whether people are competent, or are confident they can become competent, in exercising coping techniques other than drug use, or are relatively free to avoid the settings of practical action in which drugs had become integral to their perceived ability to cope (Marlatt and Gordon 1985).

Lee Robins's (1993) findings regarding the very low level of relapse to heroin use among returning Vietnam veterans; Dan Waldorf's (1983) and Patrick Biernacki's (1986) findings of the commonly experienced association of recovery from addiction with removal from the types of settings and associates that had constituted one's practical contexts of drug use; and the widely recognized recovery advantage had by addicts with comparatively wider ranges of coping skills and what Waldorf, Reinarman, and Murphy (1991, 10) call a "stake in conventional life" each suggest that drug use is often a more or less setting-specific coping technique that does not, as Lindesmith argued, *automatically* generalize to the whole of a person's life activities. The propensity of former users to experience strong visceral compulsions to use primarily when confronted with situations reminiscent of their old drug-using settings and associates (Childress et al. 1992) supports the conclusion that visceral drug craving is often triggered not by stress or discomfort in general but by the prereflective, though eminently meaningful, lived experience of former drug-using settings and associates and the practical demands they are tacitly perceived to entail.

Taken together, these empirical findings support the praxiological approach to understanding drug use and drug-induced experiences I have offered here. Drug use and drug-induced experiences are often deeply meaningful (if, by no means, always enjoyable) for those who undertake them. However, to fully comprehend the depth of those meanings, we must transcend the view that they amount to no more than linguistic interpretations that are projected over brute physical sensations by disembodied, cognitively constituted selves. In place of this view, I have argued we should begin to appreciate that much of that meaning is comprised in and derives from the prereflective, perceptual concomitants of people's tacitly embodied competencies for using drugs to meet the practical demands they perceive to make up their lives.

Incidentally, by showing how many different patterns of drug use could conceivably come to be experienced by drug users as beyond their control, this praxiological approach to the meaning and social learning attendant to drug use and drug-induced experience also avoids what Robin Room (1983, 55–62) has called the problem of "entitativity" faced by disease theories of addiction. Unlike disease theories, the praxiological rubric I have outlined here does not demand that we account for the vast range of patterns in which drug problems actually occur as consequences of a single disease entity like "alcoholism." Most importantly, it preserves the epistemological gains that Lindesmith's classic theory made by introducing meaning and social learning as crucial components of the addiction process while overcoming the mind-body dualism that has encumbered sociological research on drug use and experience for the better part of a century.

4

"OUT THERE"

The Ecology of Addiction in
Drug Abuse Treatment Discourse

Over the course of the nineteenth and twentieth centuries there emerged a
fairly coherent discourse regarding both the clinical characteristics of drug
addiction and the appropriate methods for its treatment (Baumohl and Room
1987; H. Levine 1978; Schneider 1978). Originally, medical professionals such
as Benjamin Rush were prominent among those who claimed addiction was
not so much a moral failing as a medical condition that demanded medical treatment. However, despite their claims-making successes, medical
professionals have often abjured the role of actually ministering to addicts
themselves. By their incursions into, and flights from, the management of
drug-related social problems, medical professionals cleared work spaces that
lay self-help groups and therapeutic communities eventually came to occupy.
These events had the effect of forging a union between two propositions on
which much of the modern addiction treatment industry is now predicated.
These propositions are: (1) drug addiction is a genuine disease marked by a
"loss of control" over one's drug use and (2) this disease can be effectively
treated through ongoing participation in a therapeutic community.

These paired propositions have been widely institutionalized in the sense that contemporary participants in addiction treatment programs throughout the world are normatively required to honor them if they are to remain in treatment. Program participants inherit these propositions as nonnegotiable institutional structures that both facilitate and constrain the kinds of activities they are expected and entitled to undertake as members of a treatment program. Given these institutionally enforced parameters, participants in addiction treatment discourse must inevitably cope with the following conceptual puzzle: exactly *how* can people who are, by definition, chronically afflicted by a disease that is beyond their own personal control be empowered to master this disease through participation in a therapeutic community? And, as a related matter, participants in drug abuse treatment discourse must be able to plausibly distinguish between the *actions* taken by program participants and the causal *effects* of their addictions.

In what follows, I suggest that these conceptual feats are accomplished, at least in part, by discursively sustaining a categorical contrast between two diametrically opposed ecologies—the recovery program itself and what I am calling the ecology of addiction.[1] Immersion in the social world of the program is held to systematically empower people to take control of their lives (Denzin 1993; Skoll 1992; Sugarman 1974; Weinberg 2000b). In contrast, the ecology of addiction, "out there," is painted as a uniformly desolate space that systematically wreaks havoc in the lives of those forced to live there. Through use of this ecological contrast, people cast themselves as accountably invested in, and capable of, recovery through participation in the treatment program but nonetheless chronically vulnerable to their addictions, which they claim are enflamed and made stronger by the temptations and frustrations of living "out there."

This analysis builds upon, and contributes to, the social problems work perspective introduced by James Holstein and Gale Miller (1993). In an effort to promote research on the *local* construction of social problems, Holstein and Miller (1993, 152) call for greater attention to the ways in which "social problems categories, once publicly established, are attached to experience in order to enact identifiable objects of social problems discourse." By giving temporal priority to the "public establish[ment]" of social problems categories, Holstein and Miller (1993) clearly indicate that social problems work is in part reliant on a stock of already accredited cultural resources. This said, though, social problems work is plainly not coextensive with the campaigns of those concerned to propound or contest the credibility of social problems categories generally. In this chapter, I show how participants in drug abuse treatment discourse effectively reconcile preestablished conceptual claims regarding the nature and treatment of their drug problems through creative use of the narrative construct I am calling the ecology of addiction. I thereby demonstrate one way in which specific instances of the social problems category "addiction" are routinely identified and addressed in therapeutic communities designed to tackle this social problem.

Settings and Methods

This analysis draws upon ethnographic materials gathered during fieldwork in three different addiction treatment programs. The first program, in which I did fieldwork for a period of four months, was a residential facility housed in one of the many privately funded Christian missions in the skid row area of downtown Los Angeles. This program served an exclusively male clientele drawn primarily from the local environs of skid row. The second program was a residential facility remotely located in the foothills above Los Angeles. This program was administered by a private nonprofit corporation but funded primarily through a joint grant from county mental health and substance abuse services. It served both women and men from all over Los Angeles County who had been dually diagnosed with co-occurring substance dependencies and serious psychiatric disorders. I spent nine months collecting data there. The third program was nonresidential but otherwise expressly modeled on the second program. It was located in Venice Beach, California, and was administered by a nonprofit research corporation as part of a federally funded study of the comparative costs and benefits of residential and nonresidential care for dually diagnosed homeless adults. I conducted fieldwork in this program for a period of seven months.

My fieldwork in each of these three programs consisted in participant-observation and unstructured interviews with both clients and counselors. I made site visits at least weekly, spending the day with program members and going through their routines with them. I regularly attended formal group therapy sessions, participated in informal and recreational activities, and privately conversed with both clients and counselors regarding their activities and experiences in the programs and related topics. All program participants were fully appraised of my status as a researcher. They were assured confidentiality and told of their right not to be included in the study. All clients and counselors in all three programs consented to participate in the research and allowed me to sit in and observe their group sessions.

Following my site visits, I wrote extensive field notes, fleshing out hastily written notes I had jotted down over the course of the day. I completed these field notes as soon as possible, normally within a few days of each site visit. In addition to approximately eight hundred pages of single-spaced typewritten field notes, I also collected written materials used in the programs and about forty hours of audiotape recordings depicting group therapy sessions, private counseling sessions, and staff meetings in the foothill program. By systematically comparing therapeutic practice in each of these three programs, I learned to distinguish narrative devices common to all three settings from those that were less common and/or unique to a given treatment program or program participant. My purpose in what follows is to both demonstrate and explain the ecology of addiction, "out there," as a narrative construct that was very commonly evident in each of the three programs I observed.

The Ecology of Addiction in Drug Abuse Treatment Discourse
"In" and "Out" in Drug Abuse Treatment Discourse

As I intimated in the introduction to this chapter, to be described as "in" the program was to be cast as a member of a community of people dedicated to helping each other overcome their addictions (Alcoholics Anonymous 2001). Conversely, when program participants relapsed it was routinely said that they had "gone out." This use of the expression "out" can be seen in the following field note excerpts,

> Janet came back onto the patio and asked how everyone was doing. Layla answered, "Lousy." Janet asked, "What's wrong?" And Ian answered, "She went out this weekend . . ." Janet looked at Layla and said, "Oh no, don't tell me. You used over the weekend?" Layla nodded sheepishly.

> After dinner Neil, Sean, and Marta talked about where Tony, Liza, Nat, and Ron were today. Neil was leaning back in his chair smoking a cigarette and in a blasé, knowing tone of voice he said, "Yesterday was check day and they're not here today. I don't think that looks too good, do you?" Sean laughed and said, "No it doesn't. You think they went out?" Neil said, "I think Liza went out and it wouldn't surprise me a bit if Nat did. In fact I'm sure that's what he did. Tony's been doin' good lately, though, but he has a hard time when he's got money. He's got a real problem with that. Ron, I dunno. I ain't sayin' they went out necessarily but I think they got their checks and they ain't thinkin' too much about the program."[2]

In the first excerpt, Janet obviously understands "went out" to specifically mean that Layla used drugs. By distinguishing "[going] out" from simply "[not] thinkin' too much about the program," Neil also makes it clear in the second excerpt that merely being AWOL from the program did not of itself qualify as "[going] out." This expression was reserved to describe only those who had relapsed. By describing Tony as "doin' good lately" but noting that he has a "hard time when he's got money," Neil indicates that the possibility of Tony's relapse did not so much reflect a lack of commitment to recovery as Tony's ongoing *struggle* with addiction. In drug abuse treatment discourse, "out," or "out there," was generally described as a space one's addiction compelled one to inhabit. It was not a space that most program members freely chose to be.[3] One can see this still more clearly in the following comments Layla shared in group therapy:

> "I'm doin' real, real bad right now. I'm feelin' real depressed. I'm havin' trouble right now stayin' clean for more than two days. . . . I hate myself for goin' out and I don't know if there's anything that can save me anymore. I'm feeling very disillusioned because I feel like I worked this program good. I worked it real hard. . . . If anybody worked this program I did and it still didn't work for me. I'm feelin' real desperate right now. . . . This last relapse was the worst I ever had and I still feel like I just want more. I think I'm gonna die out there."

Relapse was, then, routinely cast as movement from one ecological space to another. Before explaining why members of these settings were inclined to cast the reoccurrence of their disease in such terms, it will be useful to further explicate the characteristics that program participants conferred on this putative space "out there." In the following sections, I address the substance of being and/or living "out" as it was routinely represented in these settings, focusing on four major themes by which the ecology of addiction was discursively opposed to the ecology of recovery.[4] I have entitled these themes: endogenous accounts of the active addict mentality; legends of the fall; getting "clean" and being "dirty"; and the hazards "out there."

Endogenous Accounts of the Active Addict Mentality

The most critical contrast that members of my settings drew between the ecology of recovery and the ecology of addiction concerned their characteristic mentalities while inhabiting these spaces. This contrast was drawn by opposing a conscientiousness demanded by life in the program to a personal dissolution shared by those still ensconced in "the life." People in treatment were themselves described as "working a program," which, while involving a fairly vast spectrum of specific projects, basically entailed assiduous efforts to fulfill one's personal responsibilities to oneself and to others. Conversely, the mentality of the active addict was constructed fundamentally in terms of self-abandon. Whereas social scientists have often emphasized the distinctive rationality and subcultural aspects of addict behavior (Agar 1973; Finestone 1957; Lindesmith 1947; Preble and Casey 1969; Ray 1961; Stephens 1991; Sutter 1969), treatment program participants generally construed the behavior of active addicts as indicative of disease—that is, as involuntary, self-destructive, and quite beyond the pale of any sustainable cultural order.[5] In "going out," the moral and rational dimensions of the addict's temperament were held to have essentially given way to asocial pathological drives.

Simply stated, program participants generally characterized the drug-related behaviors of active addicts as involuntary and "out of control."[6] One way this was done was by painting the addicts who remained "out there" as oblivious to their own self-interest. In the following excerpt, Kyle distinguishes himself and his peers in the program from the active addicts who spent time in and around the Mission by invoking the latter's unconsciousness of (and hence their incapacity to pursue) their own personal welfare:

> "We're all on the program. At least we've begun to see. Now I've been on the program before and I relapsed before but at least I know what I need to do. Those brothers out there? They don't even know what they're doin' to themselves."

Of course, program members did not cast themselves as immune to this kind of addictive unconsciousness but as engaged in a perpetual struggle to overcome and/or prevent it. It was precisely this putative struggle with their addictions that warranted their presence in a treatment program in the first place. Sometimes the active addict mentality was cast as an inability to consider the nature and/or consequences of one's *actions*. But it was also sometimes cast as a jaded indifference to one's own *subjective state of being*. Program participants often spoke of the active addict's life as corrosive to the capacity to express how one feels or even know how one really feels:

> "When things were goin' bad for me I just said I'll take care of it and I don't need nobody's help. I might be feelin' bad and somebody comes up to me and says, 'How you feelin'?' And I just say, 'All right.' And that's

not even an answer, that's not even a feeling! What kind of feeling is 'all right,' you know? Pretty soon, I don't even know how I feel! I'm always jus' 'all right.'"

From the constructionist perspective I am taking in this chapter, the first question to ask of such accounts is not: Are they empirically valid or invalid? But, instead: What specific practical work are they doing on the various occasions of their use? (Holstein and Miller 1993). I will return to consider this question at length in the discussion section of the chapter. However, at present I wish to remain focused on how this endogenous image of the active addict mentality, a nearly perfect antithesis to the ascendant sociological image of the active addict as rational actor, was discursively linked to a distinctive type of ecological space. In the following data excerpt, Stephen finishes his account of the depravity of his life when addicted to speed by describing this period in his life as "out."

"Speed took me to the point where I was sleeping in alleyways and was eating out of garbage cans, going around talking to myself all the time. It was the only thing I ever wanted. I didn't even care if I died. I was filthy dirty. I didn't know anybody and it gave me these sores all over my body. I was a mess but I didn't even care. I didn't care if I was addicted and I didn't care if I died... Not many people have been that far out."

Clint spoke of his own asocial behavior when he was "out there in [his] addiction."

"When I was out there in my addiction I fucked over a lot of people. I mean a lot!! I used to go up to people when I was loaded, people I didn't even know and who hadn't done a fuckin' thing to me and just smack 'em as hard as I could. . . . I was crazy as hell. . . . Those were some real nasty times. It's not just me either. . . . When you're like me you drag everybody near you down with you and that's exactly what I did, my wife, my parents, my friends. I was not somebody you would ever want as a friend."

In both of these cases, active addict behavior is specifically cast as antithetical, indeed preclusive, to cohesive social attachments. Insofar as active addiction was held to consist in dissolute behavior by which social bridges were burned, there were obvious incentives to cast the space within which addiction persisted as a socially desolate one. But even further, the putative space "out there" was itself held to *promote* addictive self-abandon. This can be seen very clearly in the following excerpt. Ian begins by painting the familiar picture of the active addict as consumed with little other than survival and the acquisition of drugs. But whereas scholars since Edward Preble and John Casey (1969) have suggested this agenda fills the addict's life with a certain, albeit tragic, meaningfulness, Ian casts it more as the mind-numbing routines of a hapless automaton.

"When you're homeless your head is just in this place of always havin' to take care of business, and watch out you don't get robbed or even hurt or killed sometimes. I'm serious. And it's just like livin' that way for a while gets you so that you're always so tense and so fuckin' frustrated about everything that nothin' matters to you anymore 'cept stayin' safe and keepin' your hustle. It's like you start gettin' into a one-track mind.... People don't even want to think about what's up wit' them. All they want is that rush of good feeling and it don't matter where that rush puts 'em or what it takes to get it 'cause you're already low down as you can get anyway. People just want to deaden themselves and that's what they do."

Here, Ian very clearly links his characterization of the active addict mentality to the relentless pressures of life on the streets and concisely describes the intimate causal relationship that was routinely drawn between what I have been calling the ecology of addiction and the active addict mentality. *In sum, within the context of drug abuse treatment discourse, the self-destructive behavior of active addicts was held to be caused not only by an intrapersonal "disease" but also by the decidedly despised ecological space that was held to sustain and exacerbate that disease.* In the following sections, I briefly demonstrate three further thematic contrasts by which program members conceptually linked an image of addicted behavior as involuntary or "out of control" with the image of addiction's responsiveness to a distinctively insalubrious ecological space.

Legends of the Fall

In addition to its being specified as a space "out there," the ecology of addiction was described as a low or degraded space, a space indicative of social decline. Following AA protocol, when people entered a treatment program they generally expressed the view that they had in some way "hit bottom," meaning their life had come to seem totally unmanageable (Alcoholics Anonymous 2001).[7] This was often cast as a personal fall from grace—a loss of one's former social standing and social connectedness. However, people also routinely attributed their movement into the program to the progressive degradation of their milieu "out there." In the following excerpt, Lonni describes the events that catalyzed her decision to get into a drug abuse treatment program.

"Life on the street was just becomin' more and more crazy and dangerous. Most of the homeless people I used to hang around with would get high. . . . They was a certain amount of people that would hang together and watch out for each other. All those people started to go against each other. . . . This one girl got pissed off 'cause she couldn't get high with this guy. And so she started arguin' with me . . . and then, when I turned around, she had a knife and was talking a lot of shit."

Lonni said this incident "made me wake up and see that living on the streets is not a good idea. I thought, 'I've been homeless for almost seven months . . .' I don't even want to deal with that shit. I got tired of that shit. I said it's time to get my shit together, at least attempt to do it."

Lonni speaks of "wak[ing] up" to the need to "get [her] shit together," and in finishing with the phrase "at least attempt to do it," she indicates this will entail a conscientious struggle, in contrast to the putative somnambulism by which she remained on the streets and unresponsive to her deteriorating near-group relations. Thus the imagery of recovery as self-governed and drug life as not self-governed is again sustained. Interestingly, these accounts of the degradation of street life sometimes went beyond descriptions of descent in one's own biography and/or one's proximal milieu to more fully inclusive accounts of collective descent from an idealized past to a current state of general desolation "out there."[8] Most generic descent stories referenced a time when street life was dominated by hippies who looked out for one another. Thus Clarise said,

"The attitude out there . . . isn't the same as it used to be. Used to be you could walk down on the beach and you'd see hippies smokin' dope or doin' whatever they was doin' and they'd let you alone. They'd be doin' their thing and you just do your thing. They was homeless but nobody was scared of 'em. Now you'd have to be crazy to be on those beaches at night."

Clarise was old enough to have known street life in the sixties firsthand. But romanticized images of the sixties were also invoked by people who acknowledged not knowing if that imagery was accurate or not. In the following excerpt, Ian uses the utopian image of the sixties as a benchmark from which to trace an ongoing deterioration of street life, the last stages of which he does claim to have witnessed firsthand.

> "People don't know what it's like to be homeless now. A lot of people think it's still like the sixties you know where everybody helps each other out. I mean I wasn't around that far back so I don't know if it was ever like that but it sure as hell ain't like that now. I remember when it used to be you'd get the rockheads all hangin' out in one place and all the drunks here and all the junkies someplace else and then maybe you had a little bit of people lookin' out for each other. I mean a little bit. You know if you got somebody high then they figure they owe you one and they'd do you a favor or somethin' but even that'd only go so far. I mean you still got ripped off a lot even then. But now there ain't even none of that anymore. Everybody just lookin' out for themselves and nobody can't do nothin' for nobody else. Nobody trusts anybody and nobody can be trusted. People rip off anyone; it don't matter who you are. It's pure shit. I used to use behind that shit all the time 'cause I just couldn't take it."

Here, Ian uses an account of collective descent into a quasi-Hobbesian order to indicate that his drug use was a product of defeat ("I just couldn't take it") and not deliberate or rational adjustment. The phrase "I couldn't take it" reflects a very different vocabulary of motives (Mills 1940) than "using drugs seemed sensible given my dire circumstances." Hence, drug use is held to reflect an environmentally induced relinquishing of self-control rather than a deliberate exercise of self-control. The excerpts in this section variously demonstrate how program members described the ecology of addiction in terms of decline from a higher, more humane social order. Sometimes this decline was cast in solely personal terms. But it was often also cast as a collective fall suffered by the bulk of those with whom one shared "the life." In contrast to the involuntary fall that delivered one over to addiction, recovery was cast as a laborious ascent from the depths (see also Marvasti 1998). While immersion in the ecology of the program could empower one to accomplish this ascent, it could not completely relieve one of the inevitable personal struggle that "getting clean" entailed.

Getting "Clean" and Being "Dirty"

Another salient feature of the ecology of addiction in drug abuse treatment discourse was its association with dirt, in opposition to the cleanness characteristic of recovery.[9] When one was known to be "in" the program they were commonly described as "getting clean." Conversely, when blood or urine tests indicated recent drug use, those tests were described as "dirty." The affinity of cleanliness with recovery and dirtiness with the drug addict's life was commonly manifest in a variety of other ways too. In the following excerpt, Clarise, a counselor, tells of her efforts to work with Del on his grooming.

"I'm trying to get him to cut his hair, shave regularly, clean his clothes—I think those things are a real important part of getting into a recovering lifestyle. Once they start caring a little more about how they look that's a real good sign that they're taking the program to heart. People may be coming regularly but if they continue to look like they're homeless and don't really take care of their appearance I can't help thinking they aren't bringing a lot of what they get in the program out with them when they leave."

Findings of an affinity between dirtiness and drug addiction were by no means limited to counselors on staff. In the following excerpt, Charlie struck a chord with many of his peers when he opened a group therapy session with a lament regarding a recent encounter with a "pan-hassler" (an aggressive panhandler). After recounting the incident to the group, he continued as follows:

"These people don't care about keepin' clean or keepin' any kind of self-respect about themselves. I'll tell ya, stayin' clean and healthy and keepin' my clothes lookin' all right is important to me. If you don't try and distinguish yourself from the scum then you'll turn into the scum. If you don't try and get yourself outta the gutter you'll become part of that gutter. And that's what a lot of these people out there are. They don't got no principles. They don't demand anything from themselves." Mack laughed and added, "They'd literally kill their own grandmother to get a hit." Charlie said, "Yep, it's all about the drugs. That's all it's about. People don't care about anyone or anything. They have no respect for themselves, no respect for other people, and no respect for their environment." Mack, Del, and Clarise were nodding fiercely in agreement. Others were also doing so occasionally.

In this passage, Charlie opposes his own conscientious efforts to "[stay] clean and healthy" to the profligate dirtiness, degradation, and amorality of "these people out there." Charlie seems to suggest that cleanliness flows from deliberate effort, dirtiness mere dissolution. Moreover, by equating them with "scum" and the "gutter," Charlie clearly invokes a close relation between a degraded space "out there" and its degraded inhabitants. The narrative linkage of this general degradation and addiction in particular can be clearly seen in Mack's taking up Charlie's lament with an unprecedented invocation of drug use ("they'd literally kill their own grandmother to get a hit"). Evidently Mack understood Charlie's complaint as one specifically about addicts, and indeed Charlie confirms Mack was correct in his next remark ("Yep, it's all about the drugs"). Once again, in its ascribed affinity to dirtiness, drug use is here held to simultaneously reflect the feral influence of a space "out there" as well as personal lapse and dissipation rather than self-governed activity.

The Hazards "Out There"

Beyond descriptions of oblivion, descent, and dirtiness, accounts of the ecological space "out there" tended to depict a doleful world fraught with myriad emotional and physical hazards. In vivid contrast to the trust, compassion, and communal solidarity ascribed to the world of the recovery community, program participants claimed overwhelmingly to have feared and/or distrusted those with whom they had shared the street. Even when they did socialize with others, members claimed they were careful not to become close. The distinction between "friends" and "acquaintances" was very commonly invoked in each of the three programs (see also Rosenbaum 1981, 57). In the following passage from a group therapy session, Claire, a counselor, chided Neil about his supposed popularity.

> "You got a million friends, right, Neil?" Neil said, "I do?" Claire said, "Yeah. Don't you? I thought you did. You talk about a lot of the people you know—" Neil interrupted, "Well I might know a lot of people but they ain't my friends. Those are acquaintances. There's a difference!" [Laughs.] The other clients laughed in recognition of the importance of this distinction. Neil continued, "I have a lot of acquaintances but I wouldn't call any of 'em my friends."

A fairly obvious result of this pervasive distrust was that the awful loneliness of living "out there" became a recurring theme in drug abuse treatment discourse. In the following field note excerpt, Lee gives a moving account of his loneliness, indicating its relation to both his drug use and his assessment of those with whom he shared the streets.

> "I've had periods in my life when I was really lonely, really lonely like when I decided to bum it last time and those were bad times . . . 'cause I

didn't know anybody and I couldn't meet anybody. That was the worst part about bein' homeless [*laughs*]. It's funny too 'cause I used to always go and sit on a bench out there in Palisades Park and there was this other homeless guy who used to sit across from the bench I sat on and one time he came over to talk to me but I said, 'Hey, I don't wanna talk to you, get outta here.'" Claire asked, "Why'd you do that?" Lee replied, "I don't know why. Maybe I thought I was better than him unconsciously or somethin'. Maybe I was scared he was gonna con me or rip me off. I dunno." Tanya nodded and laughed in agreement. Neil also nodded in recognition of the sentiment Lee was expressing. Lee spoke again, "I get lonely, though. It's bad. That's the worst feeling I know, loneliness. That's always when my worst depressions would set in and when I got depressed that was when I'd relapse. You know you just start thinkin' like nobody cares so you say 'Why should I care? I don't care either.'"

Similar to Ian's report, in this account Lee attributes his relapses to the demoralization, fear, and loneliness he suffered while living out. Relapse is thus cast not as a deliberate act of self-control but as a relinquishing of self-control in the face of overwhelmingly adverse circumstances ("you just start thinkin' like nobody cares so you say 'Why should I care? I don't care either'"). In addition to being characterized by loneliness, life "out there" was also commonly described as disorderly and dangerous. Danny put it this way after Eve asked him about his motivation to get clean:

Eve asked, "Do you want to get clean now?" Danny answered, "Well sort of. I don't know really. I'm sick of all the bullshit." Claire asked, "What bullshit?" and Danny said, "You know the street stuff: getting robbed, getting beat up, losin' your stuff all the time, bein' dirty all the time."

People represented the ecology of addiction as fraught with predators and the threat of harm. But, as I have said, it was not simply that living "out there" forced one to contend with the prospect of being robbed, hurt, or killed. Of course, those prospects were described as ever present but, even further, the predatory and licentious nature of the street-addict scene was cast as infectious. According to program participants, drugs were only one element of a much wider set of circumstances that forced people into "the life." Poverty, homelessness, and unemployment were all given their due as well (see also Rosenbaum 1981; Wacquant 1998), as were the many disastrous consequences of the war on drugs (see also Reinarman and Levine 1997). Indeed, it cannot be overstated how much the continuing legacy of drug prohibition and criminalization has yielded the miseries that program participants associated with life "out there." The condition of living among others "out there" and having to compete with them for the scarce resources necessary to sustain one's own survival was often given particular emphasis. According to Del,

> "Those people out there are dangerous, they're rude, they're selfish, they're diseased a lot of 'em and they don't care about anything. They've seen it all and nothing affects them anymore. They're numb. They ain't got no sympathy for anyone 'cause they don't feel like anyone's got any sympathy for them. You see it all the time. People in the food line lyin' about how they got a family they gotta bring stuff back to so they can get more than their share. They ain't got no family they're just selfish dirty dogs who wanna get as much as they can get and they don't care about nobody else. That's the streets. That's just what ya gotta contend with every day. Ain't nothin' new about it. I been dealin' with that for years. You just gotta learn how ta deal with it." Charlie said, "Sometimes it really gets under my skin."

As Charlie's remark indicates, program members by no means cast themselves as immune to the pressures of life "out there." This is also evident in the following field note excerpt, wherein Rickie comments on his having been accused by some of his peers in the program of "acting like a dope fiend" and "having an attitude."

> "I don't know why they think that. I know I had an attitude out on the streets, but ya had to have an attitude if you wanted to survive, you know? Up here ain't no reason to do that stuff. . . . Out there's a different story, though. You know you get burned and you burn somebody back, you know? That's just the way it is on the streets. After a while you lose your twenty [dollar bill] so many times you say, 'I ain't gonna be the only one who's losin'!' . . . It's crazy out there. Nobody trusts nobody. I didn't know nobody and I didn't trust nobody enough to be runnin' with him as a partner. He'd be the dude that gets me, you know?"

Here, Rickie acknowledges an "attitude" but insists that it is drawn out of him by conditions "out there" and is decidedly not an enduring feature of his personal temperament. As he says, in the program there "ain't no reason to do that stuff." The ecology of recovery cultivated in the treatment program is thus held to free one from the practical compulsion they might otherwise feel to "act like a dope fiend." But given the ever-looming prospect of a return to life "out there," people described themselves as "trying to change" but nonetheless eminently susceptible to the challenges that this distinctively dysfunctional ecological space posed to their recovery. When confronted by the world "out there," people claimed to feel powerfully drawn toward comporting themselves in ways that were responsive to that world, even if these responses were recognized as ultimately self-destructive. Living "out" or "out there" was to live under crazy, violent, and capricious circumstances. In other words, the ecological space indicated by reference to "out" or "out there" was held to powerfully entice, if not relentlessly compel, its inhabitants to live savagely and licentiously for the moment and anticipate betrayal by anyone. I will now discuss the specific utility of this narrative construct in drug abuse treatment discourse, and hence its persistence in this particular type of social problems work.[10]

Discussion

Students of the history of social problems theory will no doubt have observed in many of the foregoing accounts a certain affinity with what I call sociogenic personal deficit theories—theories such as social pathology, social disorganization (Faris and Dunham 1939), disaffiliation, undersocialization (Pittman and Gordon 1958; Straus 1946), and Richard Cloward and Lloyd Ohlin's (1960) famous double-failure theory of addiction. Much like these sociological theorists, participants in my programs seemed to condemn certain types of drug-related practices as pathological and to explain these practices as in part responsive to the dysfunctional ecological environments within which they are held to develop. Though their substantive affinity is real, it is critically important that we carefully distinguish the foregoing accounts from those given by sociologists. Why? Because in their accounts of addictive drug use, participants in drug abuse treatment discourse and sociologists are engaged in entirely different sorts of work. Whereas participants in drug abuse treatment discourse are using these accounts in a primarily therapeutic context to do primarily therapeutic work, sociologists use such accounts in an academic context to do scientific work.

While it is fair enough to criticize scientific theories because they are logically muddled or inadequate in light of extant data, such complaints are somewhat off point if they are made of accounts being used to do something other than scientific description (Bogen and Lynch 1993, 214; Bourdieu 1990). We must not forget that program participants were not themselves doing social science, nor were they particularly concerned to reconcile their accounts with social scientific theory. They were concerned to solve what they viewed as their own problems in living. This said, however, it may still be useful for present purposes to briefly compare their accounts with those given by social scientists. The ethnographic literature on homeless street life, "street addict culture," and "bottle gangs" is fairly abundant, with convincing critiques of the starkly pathological images found in the writings of sociogenic personal deficit theorists. Largely due to ethnographic critiques, most social scientists have long since abandoned sociogenic personal deficit theories as better documents of researcher preconceptions than careful empirical analyses (Mills 1943; Wiseman 1970). Likewise, then, this literature strongly suggests that, as a strictly scientific matter, the desolate images of life "out there" painted by clients in my settings were at least selective descriptions of street life and quite probably also somewhat exaggerated. Simply stated, then, the ethnographic literature provides very good scientific reasons for us to wonder why people in treatment programs so consistently describe not only their own personal drug habits but the whole drug scene in such profoundly disparaging terms.

Let me now return to my suggestion that we focus our attentions on the two propositions I described in the introduction to this chapter as foundational to contemporary drug abuse treatment discourse: (1) drug addiction is a genuine disease marked by "loss of control" over one's drug use and (2) this disease can be effectively controlled through ongoing participation in a therapeutic community. As mentioned earlier, participants in my research settings inherited these paired tenets as nonnegotiable institutional structures. To the extent they sought to remain as participants in good standing in these settings, their actions were inevitably both facilitated and constrained by the organizationally enforced requirement that both tenets be honored. This meant that participants in these programs inevitably had to work out exactly *how*, despite being always prone to enslavement by their addictions, they were also capable of being empowered to master their "disease" through ongoing participation in a therapeutic community. It is in light of this institutionally enforced conceptual puzzle that the distinctive utility of the narrative construct I have been calling the ecology of addiction can be most clearly understood.

Let us begin with the first tenet. The idea that drug addiction is a bona fide "disease" historically arose and has been sustained precisely because it gives conceptual semblance to the notion that certain types of drug-related troubles reflect sufferers' "loss of control" over their personal behavior (H. Levine 1978). This has in turn provided, by far, the most politically effective means for legitimating specifically *therapeutic* approaches over punitive approaches to solving drug-related social problems (Baumohl and Room 1987; Musto 1987; Wiener 1981). Quite clearly, generic claims on behalf of "the disease theory of addiction" have been crucial in campaigns to promote therapeutic interventions at the level of public policy. But generic claims regarding the nature of drug problems do not determine how concrete instances of these problems are identified in practice (Holstein and Miller 1993; Loseke 1999). To use the disease theory of addiction to foster solutions to the problems of particular people, one must be able to plausibly identify the *symptoms* of addiction—that is, the specific personal events held to have been caused by this disease. Of course, this is not only true of addiction. This problem is but one instance of the type/token problem that is encountered by both medical and nonmedical diagnosticians of all diseases.

However, addiction is a very odd case of this problem in the following respect. Participants in drug abuse treatment discourse must plausibly attribute to a disease agent segments of personal behavior that at first blush often appear quite subtly adjusted to the social worlds in which alleged addicts live. In other words, the types of events that are held to qualify as symptoms of the disease *addiction* often look a good deal more like rational human conduct than do the types of events held to qualify as symptoms of other diseases. This can be seen in the following field note excerpt. Here, Lee explains why he had come to California and then immediately diagnoses that explanation as symptomatic of addiction. This remark was made without the slightest hint of irony or sarcasm:

> "It's warmer out here. That's the main thing. I was sick of being homeless in New York. New York is a shitty place to be homeless. It's too damn cold there. But I guess that's thinking like an addict."

It is in light of talk like this that we may begin to understand the allure that images of a distinctive ecology of addiction have for participants in drug abuse treatment discourse. Though driven by fundamentally asocial appetites rather than rational self-interest or any other specifically cultural endowments, the behavior of the active addict is nonetheless regarded as often subtly adjusted to an ecological niche that is more or less peculiar to addiction. By making recourse to such imagery, participants in drug abuse treatment discourse are able to fuse a sense of the addict's behavior as essentially antisocial and uncontrolled with the sense that it might nonetheless be exceptionally sly and/or well honed to the demands of "the life." This fusion of guile and disease is well illustrated in the following discussion between Clarise and Bob.

> Clarise said, "Mack relapsed." I asked what happened and she said, "Well Mack finally got his retroactive SSI check. I guess they owed him several thousand dollars or something . . ." Bob laughed sarcastically and said, "Figures, don't it? He left me holdin' the bill to the cable too. He's got all this money all the sudden and he goes off leavin' me with the bill for the cable." Clarise asked, "It was his turn?" Bob said, "Think he'd leave when it was my turn? No way. That motherfucker was goin' for all he could get. Dope fiend motherfucker is all he is." Clarise said, "We've all done things like this but that doesn't mean it ain't a shame. I thought Mack was doin' real good. I guess it just goes to show you, doesn't it, how destructive this disease can be?" Bob said, "Yep."

Given the institutionalized requirement that clients periodically construe sophisticated sequences of behavior as involuntary—caused by a disease—the image of the conniving but impetuous "dope fiend" is of considerable conceptual utility. But what of the second basic tenet of drug abuse treatment discourse? How might a disease that is, by definition, beyond the personal control of the individual sufferer be construed as somehow amenable to the control of a group of sufferers linked as a therapeutic community? Social scientists have made a variety of important contributions to explaining the therapeutic process in group settings but in doing so we have generally forsaken the view that addictions are diseases in favor of a basically rational choice model. Richard Stephens (1991, 180) is only one of the more explicit exponents of this position:

> Street addicts are generally what I would refer to as "rational actors." To a large extent, they "choose" to become street addicts. However, remember that this "choice" is conditioned by the socioeconomic circumstances in which the vast majority of addicts find themselves. The street addict role is one of only a few relatively rewarding roles open to most persons who become street addicts. Therefore, we need not "blame the victims" for choosing one of the very limited number of available roles.... If the street addict role becomes too onerous..., or if other roles can be made more attractive, most persons will abandon the street addict role.

No doubt rational choice theory does in fact go a considerable distance in *sociologically* accounting for entrées into and exits out of episodes of heavy drug use (Elster and Skog 1999). However, as a conceptual resource for participants in drug abuse treatment discourse, it is profoundly problematic. It is problematic because it compels program participants to think about their relapses, and indeed all their behavior while addicted, as having been rationally calculated. Adopting this conceptual framework summarily precludes attributing any behavior to the disease that program members use to conceptually justify their need for and entitlement to therapeutic assistance in the first place. Given their current mandate, participants in drug abuse treatment discourse must somehow reconcile the view that they can be socially empowered to overcome their drug problems with the view that those problems are indeed caused by a disease over which they have little or no personal control.

This kind of social problems work does not only require concepts that plausibly explain or justify drug-related activities; it specifically requires concepts that allow these activities to be plausibly *disowned*. It is only by plausibly distinguishing the *actions* of clients from the *effects* of their addictions that clients might be simultaneously understood as amenable to the restorative influence of a therapeutic community *and* afflicted by the disease that alone justifies and demands that therapeutic engagement. Furthermore, participants in drug abuse treatment discourse require concepts that go beyond merely providing credible justification for absolution or the disowning of past misdeeds. "Working a program" is an essentially *ongoing* exercise of anticipating and preventing the rekindling of people's putative problems with drugs, and it requires concepts that not only facilitate but actually warrant such a project in the first place.

Insofar as it is precisely the therapeutic community—the ecology of the program—that is held to possess medicinal force, simple logic dictates that whatever forces are held to possess the potential for rekindling addiction (and that alone warrant ongoing participation in the program) must be located, as it were, ecologically elsewhere. There are, then, strong organizational incentives for linking people's addictions with an unhealthful ecological space "out there," or beyond the confines of the program. These incentives stem from the distinctive practical logic of drug abuse treatment discourse—specifically, its demand that participants reconcile the view that they can be *socially* empowered to overcome their drug problems with the view that those problems are caused by a *disease*. The reality of this organizationally enforced conceptual puzzle, combined with abundant ethnographic testimony to the richly nuanced social organization of homeless street life and street drug and alcohol use, strongly suggests the following analytic conclusion: the recurrent accounts in my settings of a savage and unhealthful space "out there" flow less from participants' native familiarity with such a uniformly desolate space than from their subjective investment in the distinctive conceptual logic of contemporary drug abuse treatment discourse itself.

There is a more general, though perhaps less original, conclusion that follows from this analysis as well. The ethnographic habit of distinguishing etic and emic orientations to social phenomena, or outsider and insider perspectives, can all too easily slip into a rather more methodologically dangerous distinction between those who possess firsthand knowledge of social phenomena and those who do not. Reliance on this latter distinction will then sometimes encourage us to think of the "local knowledge" of those who presently inhabit a social world as valid knowledge and all other perspectives as variously biased and/or distorted. Hence, in the present case, one may feel compelled to argue that the descriptions I have analyzed here are somehow less valid than are those provided by people who remain active on the street drug scene. I think this would be a grave analytic mistake for two reasons.

First, though I have argued there is good reason to believe my research subjects' reports were selective and perhaps exaggerated accounts of the negative dimensions of the street drug world, they were still as much "firsthand" reports as are those offered by people who remain in that world. Second, we must be cautious about attributing too much descriptive innocence to the accounts offered by people who remain on the street. While we are now decades past the prima facie prejudice that street drug users cannot be reliable interviewees, this does not mean their accounts are ever comprehensive, nor does it mean they are pristine (see Holstein and Gubrium 1995). Description is always partial, selective, and responsive to the practical activities within which it participates. Hence, rather than seeking only to distinguish genuine truth tellers from the weavers of fictional yarns, a more methodologically sensible and theoretically fruitful course would be to locate, describe, and explain the shared activities within which, and specifically for which, description is undertaken. That is precisely what I have sought to do here.

5

THREE PROBLEMS WITH THE
ADDICTION AS AKRASIA THESIS THAT
ETHNOGRAPHY CAN SOLVE

In his justly famous intervention into the debate as to whether weakness of the will is possible, the philosopher Donald Davidson (2001, 29) wrote, "There is no proving such actions exist; but it seems to me absolutely certain that they do." I agree. The fact that there is no proving, in Davidson's strict sense, that such actions exist, though, advises a more inclusive and pragmatic assessment of the value of adopting this interpretation of action in any given instance. In what follows, I take a broad look at the value of interpreting addiction, in particular, as a form of weakness of the will, and/or akrasia. I then consider three problems that arise from adopting the specific views defended by those who have explicitly made the case for this thesis as well as some of their less explicit fellow travelers. To be clear, I am certain that some drug problems do in fact exhibit all the characteristics I myself would associate with akrasia. However, the thesis that addictions ought to be generally understood as a form of akrasia seems to me to be vulnerable in certain important respects.

The first section of the chapter provides an overview of the current state of debate surrounding the "addiction as akrasia" thesis. The work of the distinguished clinical psychologist Nick Heather is given pride of place as it is he who has provided by far the most methodical, comprehensive, and incisive defense of this thesis. However, the work of other important contributors to this and related debates in the addiction science literature is also critically considered. The chapter then elaborates on three problems with this thesis as it is currently formulated that I believe can be effectively addressed ethnographically.

The first problem is that this thesis too often posits the rational unity of properly functioning or healthy self-control as an integrated source of evaluation and volition. There are very good reasons to believe to the contrary, though, that properly functioning healthy people exhibit varying degrees of rational unity and disunity that are often explicable sociologically. The second problem is that this thesis too often posits self-control as invariably an exercise in emotional restraint, response inhibition, or delayed gratification. Once again, however, there are very good reasons to believe that self-control is also exercised through self-discovery and self-actualization, which are not so obviously opposed to emotional expression, disinhibition, and personal gratification. Finally, the addiction as akrasia thesis tends to undertheorize the intrinsic relationship between experience, evaluation, and volition and the social contexts within which these are shaped, stabilized, stimulated, and sustained. The chapter concludes with some brief reflections on the ramifications of these arguments for addiction science and treatment.

The Addiction as Akrasia Thesis

In a series of important essays, Nick Heather, sometimes with his colleague Gabriel Segal, has developed the argument that addiction is beneficially understood as a particularly extreme form of akrasia (Heather 2017, 2020; Heather and Segal 2013, 2015). Drawing selectively from each of these essays, I outline both the arguments they have made and their specific intentions in doing so. Most fundamentally, these arguments have been developed to provide philosophical "clarification regarding the conceptual foundations on which a theory of addiction should be based" (Heather and Segal 2013, 445). While the two essays by Heather and Segal remain largely agnostic regarding the best theor(ies) with which to scientifically define and explain addiction, the two essays written by Heather alone link the addiction as akrasia thesis to what are commonly called "dual process" or "dual systems" theories of addiction (Heather 2017, 2020). In this section, I attend to both the philosophical arguments concerning addiction as akrasia and the relationship Heather and others have drawn between these arguments and dual process and/or dual systems arguments concerning human decision-making generally and in the case of addiction specifically.

The core objective of these arguments is to develop a conceptual middle ground between the arguments one often finds, on the one hand, among brain disease theorists that addiction is an overwhelming or irresistible compulsion that the addict has no ability to control and, on the other hand, arguments that addiction is no more than a myth because behavior deemed addicted is, as it turns out, not scientifically distinguishable from ordinary freely chosen activities. Disease theorists can't easily provide for the fact recurrently demonstrated in psychological and social scientific studies that most behavior attributed to addictions is "incentive sensitive" (consistent with rational cost-benefit analysis) insofar as research subjects can be incentivized to abstain from the activities to which they are ostensibly addicted. Those commonly known as "choice theorists" can't easily provide for the ubiquitous tenacity of addicted patterns of behavior even in the face of sometimes severely harmful consequences. Heather is persuaded by these critiques of both received disease and choice theories of addiction and has sought, in the concept of akrasia, an intellectual path to overcoming them.

So what, then, is akrasia? Heather and Segal (2013, 447) write that "akrasia occurs when someone acts intentionally counter to his own best judgement; in these circumstances we often say that the person lacks the willpower to do what he knows or believes to be better to do." They draw heavily upon Davidson's argument in favor of the logical possibility of akrasia. Davidson defines akrasia, or what he refers to as weakness of the will or incontinent action, as follows:

In doing x an agent acts incontinently if and only if:
(a) the agent does x intentionally;
(b) the agent believes there is an alternative action y open to him and
(c) the agent judges that, all things considered, it would be better to do y than to do x. (Quoted in Heather and Segal 2013, 448)

Heather and Segal (2013) proceed to emphasize that, for Davidson, it is necessary that the agent continues to judge that it would be better to do y at the time he does x, and they follow Davidson in this requirement.[1] They then go on to formulate the philosophical problem Davidson seeks to solve in terms of reconciling three propositions:

P1 If an agent wants to do x more than he wants to do y and he believes himself free to do either x or y, then he will intentionally do
x if he does either x or y intentionally.

P2 If an agent judges that it would be better to do x than to do y, then
he wants to do x more than he wants to do y.

P3 There are incontinent actions.

Davidson's solution is predicated on a distinction between the *conditional*
akratic judgment that it would be better to do y than to do x, all things considered—that is, "relative to all facts, beliefs and values he thinks relevant to the
decision" (Heather and Segal 2013, 449)—and the *unconditional*, or strictly
logical, judgment that it would be better to do y than to do x, for which there
can be no exceptions. Because incontinent agents predicate their actions on
conditional rather than unconditional judgments, there is, philosophically
speaking, no logical contradiction. Because the conditional judgment is not
absolute (it may well ultimately prove wrong), it falls short of logically compelling the agent to act on its basis. However, Davidson argues, it remains the
case that while the incontinent agent has not behaved illogically, he has nonetheless behaved irrationally. As Heather and Segal (2013, 450) put it, "the irrationality stems from the fact that the agent's reason for doing x is, as it were,
insulated as a practical action from the better reason for not doing x." The
upshot of these arguments is that the agent, *as a rational evaluator of his own
actions*, cannot understand or rationally account for having chosen to do x.

As Heather and Segal (2013, 2015) note, this condition of having acted contrary to one's better judgment and of not understanding or being unable to rationally account for one's actions appears deeply resonant with the reports of
many putative addicts who tell us not of voluntarily "choosing" the activities
to which they are presumed addicted but of feeling alienated from and confused by their cravings to engage in these activities. This is vividly illustrated,
for example, in the following statement I observed in a group therapy session
while conducting ethnographic research in an addiction treatment program:

> I've promised myself I wouldn't use a thousand times and really meant
> it. And then I use. I mean it's like there are two sides of me. The rational
> reasonable person who knows he's gonna die if he keeps on living the
> way he is and the insane one who just doesn't care. My reasonable side
> of me can be as sure as it wants to be but when those drugs appear in
> front of me the insane one takes over and all those reasons I had not to
> use are just gone. They just disappear. And I use. It's like my mind just
> goes dead and my addiction takes over. I hate myself right afterwards

and I'm completely confused by the fact that I just used. I didn't want to but I did. It's all well and good to say you need to make a commitment but for some of us that's not enough. We need something more than that and it doesn't help for people to be all smug about how we need to make a commitment and it's all that simple.

Well-known writers on addiction such as Stanton Peele (1989) and John Davies (1992) have insisted that such accounts are not valid descriptions of the experiential reality of addiction but merely socially functional for those who provide and/or believe them. Cultures like our own, they argue, furnish people with narratives of addiction that they embrace and apply strategically to fulfill their own self-interests. I dispute neither the claim that these accounts are socially functional nor that they reflect conceptual commitments prevalent in the cultures to which putative addicts belong. What I do dispute is the claim that either of these facts necessarily forecloses on an account also being honest and/or descriptively valid (Gubrium and Holstein 2009; Haraway 1991). All accounts, including the most rigorous scientific accounts, are socially functional and reflect received conceptual commitments prevalent in the particular cultures in which they are made. Therefore, contra writers such as Peele and Davies, pointing out that an account is socially functional and culturally embedded should not be confused with a decisive refutation of either its honesty or its descriptive validity.

The addiction as akrasia thesis, and its philosophical provision for how it could possibly be that people might act intentionally counter to their own best judgment, serves better than do conventional disease theories to provide for the fact that addicted behavior is intentional behavior. People are often quite shrewd in their efforts to facilitate and fulfill their addictions. By orthodox neurological lights it is hard to see how addictive drug-using activities might be construed as symptomatic of or causally determined by a biomedical pathology precisely because they are so obviously intentional or purposive. However, unlike the addiction as ordinary rational choice thesis, the addiction as akrasia thesis also creates conceptual space for the claim that addiction is in some sense a genuine affliction over which the akratic sometimes struggles for control. As such, however, the addiction as akrasia thesis does not in its philosophical form flesh out scientifically or explain specifically what it is that subverts our better judgment or so often makes addicted behavior so unfathomable to people.

Without abandoning the premise that addictive behavior is freely chosen, the dual process or dual systems approach with which Heather (2017, 2020) and others link the addiction as akrasia thesis is intended to provide a more satisfactory scientific understanding of the phenomenology of addiction as affliction and to better explain the tenacity of addictions despite some people's concerted efforts to overcome them. This approach posits that human decision-making is based on two distinct forms of mental activity: one that is variously characterized as fast, automatic, habituated, directly responsive to external cues, impulsive, affective, unintentional, unconscious, and energy efficient; and a second that is slower, deliberative, conscious, self-directed, rational, intentional, rule-based, decontextualized, and energy inefficient. These systems are often referred to as system 1 and system 2, and I will follow this convention. The first system we are said to share with higher animals; the second is distinctly human (Evans and Frankish 2009). Heather (2017, 2020) argues that addiction reflects one type of conflict that can emerge between these two systems (see also Holton and Berridge 2013; Levy 2013). It is, then, to be clear, a case of addiction residing in the first of these systems, and the self that is afflicted invariably residing in the second. The reason addicts, *as rational evaluators of their own actions*, often cannot understand or rationally account for their addictions is that decisions based in the first system are in fact often comparatively insulated and comparatively immune to decisions based in the second.

In addition to the studies conducted by self-proclaimed dual process and/or dual systems theorists themselves (Evans and Frankish 2009; Heather 2020; Henden 2017), there is a wealth of evidence to support this approach to be found in the clinical (Garland and Howard 2018), behavioral economic (Ainslie 1992), disinhibition (Kallmen and Gustafson 1998), ego depletion (Baumeister 2003), ethnographic (Weinberg, chapter 4, this volume), neurological (Robinson and Berridge 2003), and philosophical (Levy 2013) literatures on addiction as well. For example, a large and growing literature linking clinical recovery from addiction to various mindfulness techniques is broadly consistent with dual systems theories (Garland and Howard 2018). The ethnographic data excerpt cited earlier in this chapter seems to support something like a dual systems approach, as does much of the ethnographic literature on addiction and recovery. Space constraints do not allow me to do full justice to these literatures or to the various ways in which support for a dual systems understanding of addicted decision-making can be found in them. Suffice to say that I fully acknowledge that much robust support can be found in these literatures. However, as I have said, there are also some important vulnerabilities to this approach that I believe require highlighting. It is to these that I now turn.

Is Self-Control Necessarily Rationally Coherent?

Though the addiction as akrasia thesis as supplemented by dual systems theories divides decision-making processes into two systems, it nonetheless tends to locate processes of self-control specifically in only one of these systems— system 2, the rational and deliberative one. Moreover, the rational and deliberative decision-making system is pervasively cast as capable of "all things considered" judgments predicated on conscious, decontextualized, rule-based deliberations (Henden 2017, 127). In some cases, this is cast in terms of executive function and survival relevant behavior. Sometimes, it is cast somewhat less narrowly in terms of people's long-term interests or preferences and short-term temptations, but the locus of self-control (as opposed to mere volitional choice) is invariably specified in terms of the more or less rationally coherent, holistic, and deliberative decision-making system. These arguments are often vague about exactly what expressions like "all things considered," "decontextualized," or "rational" actually mean in any given case and/or simply inconsistent with much of the scholarly literature. They often do not provide sufficiently for the manner in which type 2 decision-making processes are invariably based on foundations provided by type 1 processes (Evans 2009; Frankish 2009; Saunders and Over 2009). And, because they tend to be formulated in etic rather than emic terms, they usually result in generic specifications of addiction that can seem rather remote from the exigencies of particular people's addictions and the provision of therapeutic care. As I show in this section, ethnography can provide substantial contributions to clarifying these matters.

Let us begin with some rather high-profile firsthand accounts of the experience of addiction, those to be found in the "Big Book" of Alcoholics Anonymous (Alcoholics Anonymous 2001).[2] In addition to outlining general principles, the Big Book presents several dozen personal stories of alcohol addiction. One thing that is immediately evident about these various accounts is that in fact they are so various. The personal narratives supplied in the Big Book are not easily subsumed under a singular generic account of the reasons for people's alcohol use or the eventual problems that ensued for these people. More generally, the truly vast diversity of ways in which addictions arise in people's lives suggests it may be wise to sometimes leave aside the effort to learn the universal essence that unites them all and to conceive of the problems of addicts in terms of what the philosopher Ludwig Wittgenstein (1958) called family resemblances. We cease to search for the essence of the abstraction—addiction—that all addicts share in common. Instead, we turn ethnographically to the local details of practice within which people variously construe events as evidence of addiction. Focus shifts from addiction as such to how particular people's specific addictions are configured.

As ethnographers, we must recognize not only the commonplace that different cultural backgrounds may very well dictate different orientations to whether given activities, including drug-using activities, are or are not problematic but also that particular people may find themselves torn between conflicting values with respect to this question (Ray 1961; Room 1976). This holds for not only the first-order values by which we normally conduct ourselves but also the second-order values, or what the philosopher Charles Taylor (1989) calls the "hyper-goods" we use as standards against which to compare and coordinate our first-order values. The ethnographic literature on morality and ethics is replete with evidence that many, perhaps most, of us do not live in a coherent evaluative universe wherein "all things considered" judgments can be achieved through rationally coherent assessments or result in coherent, consistent, or stable preferences (Laidlaw 2014). This literature suggests addicts are by no means the only people who suffer chronic struggles to rationally reconcile their preferences, to set their priorities, or, more colloquially, to achieve balance in their lives. And if most of us suffer from chronic challenges in this department, perhaps it is time to refine and disaggregate our understanding of the characteristics that define particular people's selves and the specific addictions held to afflict them in light of these more ubiquitous challenges.

One element of this refinement will entail a greater recognition of the fact that how we contemplate our preferences and our "all things considered" judgments of them usually involves a complex and often fluid personal mix of emotive and intellectual considerations only sometimes more and sometimes less amenable to propositional expression, comparison, and rational reconciliation. Not only are we sometimes prone to fetishize or repress our beliefs on the kinds of psycho-emotional grounds studied by psychoanalysts, but we may also distrust or dismiss the machinations of propositional rationality on other grounds as well. Indeed, as Wittgenstein (1953) taught us, conscious, rule-based deliberations are even themselves invariably grounded in prediscursive dispositional competences forged in what he calls particular forms of life—that is, ecologically bounded fields of activity. This insight suggests that even type 2 mental processes cannot be fully "decontextualized," or disengaged from our prediscursive dispositional habits and the habitats that shape them (Brubaker 1993; Taylor 1993).

These culturally diverse forms of dispositional competence ground different forms of deliberation and evaluative priorities depending on the practical fields in and for which they are acquired, provoked, and engaged. These
deliberations and evaluative priorities may sometimes, among some people,
be subject to more general meta-level evaluations if people become for some
reason invested in the production of a more coherent ethic, lifestyle, or life
story, but the more usual pattern is that unless they overtly, persistently, and
consequentially clash, they are left to their benignly mutual irrelevance. I
possess, for example, dispositional competencies that facilitate my navigating
road traffic in a car and for composing academic papers that ground different
forms of rational deliberation and evaluative priorities. But I have never felt
compelled to rationally reconcile them to one another or to ask whether I
self-identify, all things considered, more fundamentally as a driver or an academic. I'm not sure I would know how to answer such questions even if I was
so disposed. In short, our dispositional competences are multiple, heterogeneous, and, depending on several factors to be considered here, may be more
or less rationally coherent. While they need not necessarily do so, dispositional competences may also extend beyond merely instrumental considerations of how best to succeed in particular practical contexts and into various
forms and degrees of self-identification with the practices in question. Hence,
deciding which bundle of such competences is best seen to be the locus of
a person's self-control can very often be a quite labile and dynamic matter
that, in any case, indispensably requires getting to know them personally.
Generic differentiations of type 1 from type 2 decision-making processes and
their concomitant identification of self-control invariably with the latter are
simply too rigid and too blunt to get us to the ethnographic diversity of self-
identification and self-control in what Edwin Hutchins (1995) calls "the wild."

Is Self-Control Necessarily Emotionally Repressive?

As noted in the previous section, the addiction as akrasia thesis as currently
articulated tends overwhelmingly to equate self-control with executive function and/or sticking to one's long-term interests or preferences. System 2
decision-making processes are here construed as sometimes vulnerable
to irrational short-term temptations introduced by system 1 that at times
threaten, undermine, or even, as in the case of addiction, derail our self-
control. Our fears, desires, ambitions, aspirations, hopes, and other emotional attitudes figure as motivations that in order to be made rational and

expressive of our self-control must be *rationalized* and brought to heal before our survival needs and/or long-term plans. To use the term Heather (2020) now favors, they must be regulated. This orientation to self-control is evident throughout the dual process/systems literature and in some of the most influential writings on addiction more broadly (Ainslie 1992; Baumeister 2003; Kalivas and O'Brien 2008; Levy 2005).

There can be no serious doubt that self-control is often exercised in just this way and that this manner of self-control is often evidently compromised among people with addictions. However, as the ethnographic record amply demonstrates, the argument that people universally equate their own or one another's self-control or self-government with long-term planning, impulse control, or delayed gratification is undeniably false. Not only do we freely throw caution to the wind on occasion but so too on occasion do we equate our most authentic values and self-realization with our gut instincts, spontaneous desires, and other emotional impulses and, indeed, equate the kinds of cognitive processes associated with executive function or delayed gratification with alienation from our true selves, freedom, and authentic self-control (Alasuutari 1992; Hochschild 2012; Laidlaw 2014; R. Turner 1976). On these accounts, our autonomy, freedom, or self-control is undermined rather than facilitated by the inhibitions imposed by executive functions.

If we are to more fully understand how self-control can be lost to addictions, we must seek to more fully appreciate how addictions usually arise out of nonpathological habits that are initially, and perhaps for a considerable period of time, experienced as enjoyable, life enhancing, and self-expressive rather than painful, life diminishing, or self-destructive. The Big Book presents a multitude of accounts testifying to this. For instance, "When I was drinking I was ok. I understood. Everything made sense. I could dance, talk and enjoy being in my own skin. It was as if I was an unfinished jigsaw puzzle with one piece missing; as soon as I took a drink, the last piece instantly and effortlessly snapped into place" (Alcoholics Anonymous 2001, 320).

It must always be remembered that drugs are, for most people, including those who eventually develop addictions, enjoyable and performance enhancing rather than painful and performance debilitating. Indeed, it must also be remembered that a significant majority of those who take up drug use and other potentially addictive activities never become self-destructive and that, when they do, this is always a matter of degree. It is also a matter of which people often feel deeply uncertain and ambivalent. Given the extent to which expert discourse on drug use and other potentially addictive activities is skewed toward correctional and/or therapeutic agendas, it should not be surprising to anyone that this discourse tends to minimize, and sometimes completely overlook, the fact that self-destructive engagement in such activities is, by a considerable margin, the exception rather than the rule. But as John Davies (1992, xi) has quite properly insisted, "most people who use drugs do so for their own reasons, on purpose, because they like it, and because they find no adequate reason for not doing so." If freedom, autonomy, or self-control is invariably a matter of self-regulation, or the "all things considered" rational suppression of putatively irrational temptations, it is not obvious how disinhibited and potentially (but not yet) addictive activities could figure freely, enjoyably, life enhancingly, self-expressively, and on purpose in the lives of most people who use drugs, including those who eventually develop addictions.

By exploring the myriad ways in which drugs and alcohol figure enjoyably, sometimes self-expressively or indeed even productively, and, at any rate, unproblematically in the lives of people from a range of cultures and in a range of specific cultural contexts (Douglas 1987; Heath 2012; Moore 2004; Room 1984; Singer 2012; Waldorf, Reinarman, and Murphy 1991), the ethnographic literature provides a valuable complement to the bulk of addiction research that focuses only on self-destructive activities. This literature highlights the various ways and *reasons* people come to self-identify with their drug-using practices and how these practices are inextricably bound up with a multitude of features of the specific cultural contexts within which they develop. In other words, they show us that drug-using practices are not usually experienced as threatening to our self-control but, very much on the contrary, as entirely consistent with, and as manifestly enhancing of, the satisfaction with which people conduct their lives. A better ethnographic appreciation and further investigation of this reality will provide us with a wealth of specific insights as to why particular people often seem so deeply reluctant to forgo these practices and hence why their addictions are often so tenacious.

To conclude this section and in order to flesh out this account of self-identifying with one's drug-using practices in a bit more detail, it will be useful to briefly consider the philosopher Harry Frankfurt's arguments on self-identification. According to Frankfurt, we self-identify with an element of our mental life when we are "wholehearted" with respect to it. He defines this as being "satisfied" with that element, which he further specifies as follows:

> To be satisfied with something does not require that a person have any particular belief about it, nor any particular feeling or attitude or intention. It does not require, for instance, that he regard it as satisfac-

tory, or that he accede to it with approval, or that he intend to leave it as it stands. There is nothing that he needs to think, or to adopt, or to accept; it is not necessary for him to do anything at all.... Satisfaction with one's self requires, then, no adoption of any cognitive, attitudinal, affective, or intentional stance. It does not require the performance of a particular act; and it also does not require any deliberate abstention. Satisfaction is a state of the entire psychic system—a state constituted just by the absence of any tendency or inclination to alter its condition. (Frankfurt 1999, 104)

Frankfurt (1999, 105) further argues that "satisfaction with one psychic element does not require satisfaction with any other," so his is emphatically not a theory that would seem to require a rational coherence or consistency of all those psychic elements with which we self-identify. So what, then, might he mean when he argues that despite its not requiring rational coherence or the conscious, let alone deliberate, commission or omission of any active performance, satisfaction must nonetheless be "a state of the entire psychic system" or that "insofar as his desires are entirely unreflective, he is to that extent not a person at all. He is a wanton" (Frankfurt 1999, 105–6)? This puzzle is best solved by clarifying what Frankfurt means by "unreflective." He means not inactive or unconscious, both of which self-identification may very well be, but rather reason insensitive. That is, in order to retain one's status as a person (as opposed to a mere wanton), one must remain to be seen to be amenable, at least in principle, to reasonable persuasion with respect to the psychic elements with which one self-identifies or, for that matter, with which one does not. One need not actually put these into question but one must, at least, be amenable to their reasonable interrogation.

So what does this have to do with the present argument? It suggests in the first instance that self-identification, or distinguishing those psychic elements Frankfurt calls "internal" to the self from those he calls "external"—those with which we self-identify and from which flow our own freely self-willed actions from those we find alien and from which flow constraints on, or afflictions of, our freedom and autonomy—will invariably be a matter of particular selves in all their specificity rather than the self as such as the putatively generic locus of all belief and volition. Second, one's self is here identified as those elements of our psychic life that are held expressive of our character, whether they are emotionally repressive in the name of our long-term interests or preferences or emotionally expressive of our natural and often spontaneous inclinations, including our inclinations toward the people or things we love or which give us pleasure (Moran 2002). While Frankfurt (1999) insists we must be wholehearted in our identification of those elements internal to ourselves, this is not necessarily a matter of "all things considered" rational evaluations but may also include, much more modestly, efforts to merely minimize ambivalence. Ambivalence only arises when we actually become aware of conflicts between elements of our psychic life.

There is, then, no evidence that Frankfurt believes wholeheartedness requires a comprehensive self-legislative inventory. Because by Frankfurt's account so much of that with which we are satisfied to self-identify has not been deliberatively endorsed or even consciously considered, it is implausible to attribute to him the kinds of rational coherence or consistency requirements for autonomy and selfhood defended by others (Ekstrom 2005). The most tenable interpretation of the requirement to avoid wantonness, then, is only a minimalist requirement of reason sensitivity rather than a rational coherence requirement. Autonomy, will, or self-control is exercised both through emotionally suppressive self-regulation and emotionally expressive self-revelation. Therapeutic self-exploration, discovery, actualization, and empowerment overwhelmingly attend to both dimensions of who we are and what we do.

Self-Control and Social Context

There is a ubiquitous tendency among defenders of the addiction as akrasia thesis as well as many of their fellow travelers in addiction science to assume the existence of an "ideal rationality," the normative principles of which hold universally—that is, regardless of social context. Rationality and hence self-control invariably consist in honoring or being guided by these principles. Whenever or wherever someone seems not to be guided by them, we are presented with the challenge of explaining their evident irrationality and loss of self-control. Indeed, the scholarly importance of akrasia and/or weakness of the will arguments is often explicitly predicated on precisely this assumption. While there remain lively controversies in the philosophical, psychological, and economic literatures pertaining to the specific identity of these principles, the details of these debates need not concern us here. Suffice to say these debates are largely about the causes, characteristics, and consequences of this ideal rationality and much less concerned with whether we ought to think of it as universal. The principles of rationality I have in mind include but are not limited to the normative requirements that our beliefs, intentions, and actions be coherent, consistent, and stable.

It is often said that Donald Davidson himself held this view of rationality and that it undergirds his famous arguments concerning mental holism, the principle of charity, and, in turn, via the notion of "all things considered" judgments, weakness of the will. There is certainly textual evidence for the truth of this claim. However, I think it is in need of important qualification. In his essay "Paradoxes of Irrationality," Davidson (1982) goes beyond his earlier purely descriptive account of akrasia to develop a prospective explanation for how it could come about.

> Mental phenomena may cause other mental phenomena without being reasons for them, then, and still keep their character as mental, provided cause and effect are adequately segregated. . . . To constitute a structure of the required sort, a part of the mind must show a larger degree of consistency or rationality than is attributed to the whole. . . . The idea is that if parts of the mind are to some degree independent, we can understand how they are able to harbour inconsistencies, and to interact on a causal level. . . . Recall the analysis of akrasia. . . . The way could be cleared for explanation if we were to suppose two semi-autonomous departments of the mind, one that finds a certain course of action to be, all things considered, best, and another that prompts another course of action. On each side, the side of sober judgment and the side of incontinent intent and action, there is a supporting structure of reasons, of interlocking beliefs, expectations, assumptions, attitudes and desires. (Davidson 1982, 300)

In this essay, presumably because its central task was to engage with Freudian thought and, more specifically, to explain the possibility of irrationality, Davidson seems to focus on formulating this partitioning of the mind as a segregation of its rational and irrational components (though he explicitly distinguishes this division from that between Freud's conscious and unconscious mind). If indeed his intention was confined to partitioning a singular "sober" agent from an "incontinent" one, we might very well want to insist that with his philosophy of mental holism, Davidson invariably identifies self-control with that mental structure exhibiting the greatest conformity with a universal concept of ideal rationality. However, in a note he provides the following further specification of his position:

> Here as elsewhere my highly abstract account of the partitioning of the mind deviates from Freud's. In particular, I have nothing to say about the number or nature of divisions of the mind, their permanence or

aetiology. I am solely concerned to defend the idea of mental compartmentalization, and to argue that it is necessary if we are to explain a
common form of irrationality. I should perhaps emphasize that phrases
like "partition of the mind," "part of the mind," "segment" etc. are misleading if they suggest that what belongs to one division of the mind
cannot belong to another. The picture I want is of overlapping territories. (Davidson 1982, 300)

That Davidson appears agnostic as to the "number or nature of divisions
of the mind," that he casts compartmentalization as necessary to explaining a
common form of irrationality but not obviously *confined* to the explanation
of irrationality, and that these territories need not be mutually exclusive but
are instead "overlapping" suggest that Davidson was at least open to an occasional degree of vagueness, equivocality, and/or instability in our judgments
as to which territory was best understood as the locus of self-control and/or
"all things considered" judgments in any given case. In his highly Davidson-
ian discussion of Sigmund Freud and moral reflection, Richard Rorty (1991,
151) quotes Philip Rieff's reference to "Freud's egalitarian revision of the traditional idea of a hierarchical human nature" wherein self-control is invariably identified with our "higher" rational nature and set against our passions.
Rorty (1991, 152) argues that Freud "gave us a vocabulary that lets us describe
all the various parts of the soul, conscious and unconscious alike, . . . as equally
plausible candidates for 'the true self.'" Rorty (1991, 155) continues, "I want to
focus on the way in which Freud, by helping us see ourselves as centerless,
as random assemblages of contingent and idiosyncratic needs, rather than as
more or less adequate exemplifications of a common human essence, opened
up new possibilities for the aesthetic life. He helped us become increasingly
ironic, playful, free, and inventive in our choice of self-descriptions."

Rorty's attention to the rich variety of possibilities we enjoy in our choice
of self-descriptions allows us to better appreciate the implications of Davidson's views on mental compartmentalization. By Rorty's reading, Davidson
probably didn't (and would have been wrong to) believe that rational requirements like coherence, consistency, and stability were universal criteria
with which to identify selves and self-control generically. It should also be
recalled here that Davidson's principle of charity was plainly not a principle
he thought was applied exhaustively and acontextually, for its own sake, to all
the mental contents with which people self-identify. Instead, its application
was driven in the first instance by an applicant's desire to get on with their
lives in ways they find satisfying in the Frankfurtian sense and in ways that

allow them to cooperate with others in their lives with whom they feel they must, should, or would like to cooperate. The coherence we find in our own and each other's minds, then, tends to be anchored social contextually—that is, in the various forms of life within which we participate and which variously (and, to a considerable extent, discontinuously) make salient particular beliefs, intentions, values, and the practical dispositions or competences on which these are grounded.

When we speak of holism in this context, then, it is crucial that we recognize we are usually referring to a holism bounded by inductive considerations of what might conceivably be relevant to particular, collectively orchestrated practical projects and decidedly not the much more inclusive holism suggested by invocations of type 2 decision-making processes—that is, a universal, wholly decontextualized, rule-based, and consciously deliberated holism. Moreover, the partitions Davidson wrote of insulating various regions of our mental activity should not be understood as confined to partitions between the rational and irrational. Instead, they also extend to the porous boundaries we tacitly experience between the ecological contexts within which we acquire and incorporate our own particular region-specific repertoires of dispositional competences. In short, whether or not the relations between elements of our mental life figure as reasons or as unreasoned causes of what we do is not only a matter of distinguishing rational from irrational motivations but of distinguishing context-specific rationalities as well.

This can be seen in the following ethnographic field note excerpt, taken in a staff meeting of an out-patient recovery program mandated to serve homeless and precariously housed clients suffering from addiction and a concurrent major mental illness. In this case, a client, Layla, had dropped out of the program and was accumulating insurmountable debts using crack cocaine.[3] She was contacted by a counselor but resisted this counselor's efforts to place her into an inpatient recovery setting. In the absence of mitigating factors, counselors normally regarded such resistance as irrational and evidence, more specifically, of the insurmountable hold clients' addictions had over them. However, in this case there were mitigating circumstances and, despite the putative severity of Layla's relapse, her resistance was interpreted as a reasoned rational choice rather than a causal effect of her crack addiction: "She's resisting it because she doesn't want to lose her apartment. You know she moved into that apartment next to her parents' place, and it's kind of a good situation for her. If she goes into inpatient treatment she's afraid she'll lose her place. I can understand how she feels. She's in a tough situation."

In this excerpt, knowledge of Layla's practical circumstances beyond the realm of treatment and recovery led a counselor to rationalize her resistance to inpatient treatment as strategically motivated by practical circumstances rather than as evidence of the causal force of her addiction. However, more commonly, the immediate practical demands of participating in a recovery program overrode whatever judgments might be based on practical circumstances clients faced outside the program. Thus, another counselor in the same program elaborated on her difficulty getting Del to improve his personal hygiene and Neal to obtain false teeth: "People may be coming regularly, but if they continue to look like they're homeless and don't really care about their appearance, I can't help thinking they aren't bringing a lot of what they get in the program out with them when they leave. I'm working with Neal to get his teeth again for the same reason. He looks awful without his teeth. I don't think looking like that can do anything for his self-image and self-esteem."

Del, though, claimed to regard his lax personal hygiene as an exercise in personal competence and a survival tactic while living homeless, mentioning to me later that he was more likely to be robbed if he looked better. Neal said essentially the same thing, that he fit into the homeless street scene better without his dentures and this kept him out of trouble. We can see in these examples the contingency, fluidity, and indeed contestation that is often evident in determinations of whether particular people's actions are reasoned and self-governed or comparatively unreasoned and hence quite possibly evidence of the causal force of their addictions. In Layla's case, we might want to say Davidson's principle of charity was very obviously at work. However, the cases of Del and Neil are more complicated. While their counselor was evidently devoted to helping them elevate their self-image and self-esteem and, by implication, their self-control, they themselves felt this effort to empower them, guided by a well-known standard of recovery culture (foster clients' self-respect), could not be reconciled with the tactics they considered necessary to managing life on the streets. Here, the question of which rationality should be seen to be the true locus of their self-control was not nearly so clear. There seems to have been a clash between the standards of rationality characteristic of the recovery program and the standards conducive to remaining safe on the streets.

Concluding Remarks

According to the addiction as akrasia thesis as it is currently formulated, addiction science must necessarily aspire to produce universal theoretical findings regarding such things as the self, self-control, the will, autonomy, freedom, and addiction itself. Whatever value addiction science may bring to the field of therapeutics is in this light cast uniformly in terms of the aptness of these universal models to the needs of caregivers and receivers. The thesis of this chapter is that we might instead begin with ethnographic research on the diverse and particular needs of caregivers and receivers in the myriad settings in which recovery is a concern. The insights so gleaned might then be used to interrogate the limitations of received universal models and thereby enrich our scientific understanding of addiction and recovery through a refinement and disaggregation of our knowledge of the various ways that these become manifest in the wild.

This is by no means a rejection of the aspirations of universalist addiction science as such but rather a call to recognize that ethnography provides a distinctively robust but particularist alternative to the conduct of addiction science that can incisively supplement universalism. Philosophers such as Ludwig Wittgenstein, Donald Davidson, Harry Frankfurt, and Richard Rorty have given us powerful philosophical justifications and philosophical resources with which to clarify and accomplish this kind of particularist inquiry. More specifically, the preceding arguments are entirely consistent with Davidson's views on both akrasia and mental compartmentalization. Ethnography is perhaps the best, if not the only, method of empirical inquiry for illuminating the reality of just how people in practice collectively orchestrate determinations that they themselves, and one another, have acted for reasons of their own, as a matter of self-government, or have been caused to do something by an addiction that exists external to that self (Weinberg 2005). It is for this reason I have cast this intervention not as a critique of the addiction as akrasia thesis but rather as an effort to bring ethnography to bear on the solution of three specific limitations and/or vulnerabilities one now finds in the literature. From these philosophers and a wealth of important ethnographic work on drug use, addiction, and everyday ethical practices we have learned that self-control is a matter of not only rational self-regulation but also self-expression and that it extends to the exercise of freedom in all its guises. If we are to more fully understand addiction, we must understand that it poses a threat not only to our self-regulation but also to our freedom more generally conceived.

6

TOWARD AN ECOLOGICAL

UNDERSTANDING OF ADDICTION

Defenders of the brain disease paradigm have consistently emphasized the importance of defending a medical frame for drug problems, not only because they believe the best research suggests the scientific truth of this frame but because they believe it is politically and culturally indispensable that we define addiction as a disease if it is to be met with compassion rather than retribution (Leshner 1997). In this chapter, I take a closer look at this claim as well as the claims of those who oppose it. I assess the extent to which received science has or has not provided a compelling warrant for therapeutic care over moral blame. As will be seen, I have reservations regarding some of the disease camp's arguments and some of the arguments of those who oppose the disease paradigm, and I seek to provide a path forward in what I am calling an ecological understanding of addiction.

I argue that, while it has long been widely accepted that social contexts play an important role in the initiation, entrenchment of, and recovery from problematic drug use, the mechanisms through which contexts are currently said to influence addictive behavior are invariably cast as mere cues, "secondary reinforcers," or as diverse types of incentives and disincentives that induce addicts to behave as they do. As a consequence, addiction gets theoretically construed as either a fundamentally neurological matter with only ancillary and arbitrary links to social context or as the product of social contextually informed cost-benefit analyses. As I show, in both cases addiction is ultimately construed as little more than a harmful and recurrent lust for immediate self-gratification. But if addiction is essentially just a recurrent form of lust, then on what grounds shall we argue that addicts are in need, and deserving, of compassion and therapy as opposed to mere disincentives or punishment? In this chapter, I describe one particularly robust way that the influence of context on addiction can be explained without thereby weakening the warrant for therapeutic care.

Some Historical Context
From the Critique of Luxury to the Triumph of Liberalism

As was seen in chapter 2, during the eighteenth century Christian reformers and others joined forces in opposition to both the errant indulgences of the crown and court and the licentious pursuit of profit they observed among the increasingly ubiquitous men of commerce. This was particularly true after the so-called gin craze that swept England in the early eighteenth century. By the time Benjamin Rush and Thomas Trotter lent their own authority to the notion that habitual drunkenness is a genuine disease—in the late eighteenth and early nineteenth century—the general contours of their arguments had become all but commonplace among Christian intellectuals and civic republican patriots. These kinds of arguments were also well rehearsed among early social scientists. Both Karl Marx and Émile Durkheim indicted the growth of capitalism as behind the increasing tendencies of people to become enslaved by their appetites. It was industrial capitalism, they argued, that lured people from an orientation to consumption bound to the satisfaction of needs to one of limitless self-destructive insatiability. In his *Economic and Philosophical Manuscripts*, for example, Marx (1978, 93) wrote of capitalism: "*excess* and *intemperance* come to be its true norm." Because capitalism thrives best when people continue to consume and to spend well beyond what they need, it systematically intensifies our appetites beyond our capacities to ever really fulfill them and perhaps, in more extreme cases, to even survive them. For his part, Durkheim wrote of capitalism unleashing an "insatiable will" that thrust us into an infinite and unregulated pattern of desire that ultimately causes more existential angst, or anomie, than personal fulfillment (Reith 2019).

As the modern era matured, though, liberal institutions and sentiments grew ascendant and have largely eclipsed the kinds of concerns expressed by the likes of Marx and Durkheim. Fears about the tendency of city life to kindle unbridled and self-destructive passions have increasingly come to seem hopelessly old-fashioned, quaint, narrow-minded, and priggish. Not only has liberalism largely won the day in the Western, and particularly the American, context, but it has grown so successful in capturing our imaginations that many now take liberalism to be less a theoretical outlook or moral system than the universal and natural order of things. As the distinguished historian Joyce Appleby (1992, 1) has noted, "What in Europe formed the program for a political party became in the United States a description of reality." Many liberal principles have become so enshrined in our modern Western institutions and sentiments that they are now virtually beyond debate. Few, for example, would wish to take issue with the claims that "human nature manifests itself universally in the quest for freedom. Political self-government emanates from individual self-control. Nature has endowed human beings with the capacity to think for themselves and act in their own behalf. This rational self-interest can be depended on as a principle of action. Free choice in matters of religion, marriage, intellectual pursuits, and electoral politics is the right of every individual" (Appleby 1992, 1).

The utilitarian conception of the self as autonomous happiness maximizer has, then, become far and away the most influential of the modern era and remains fundamental to the liberal creed. But, as we have seen, in this liberal view there can be no distinction between what we desire and what we consider good because our only measure of goodness is in fact what we desire. This liberal conception of self-government and rationality makes distinguishing freedom from the pursuit of what we desire axiomatically impossible and, hence, conceptualizing the idea of enslavement by one's desires—that is, addiction—equally impossible. It is the rise of liberalism to a position of self-evident common sense that has largely framed contemporary addiction science as a debate between those who construe addiction as a biological affliction of our liberal freedoms and those who see addiction as really little more than a concept with which to pathologize the liberal freedoms exercised by some deemed "others."

While the importance of social context was widely taken for granted in addiction science throughout the nineteenth century, more exclusively biological and psychological understandings slowly displaced this research toward the close of that century. The public debate turned decidedly away from reforming or therapeutically caring for those with addictions and toward prohibition and criminal punishment. Addiction science, to the extent it survived, was engulfed by this more general cultural trend and was largely subordinated to criminal justice agendas. Accordingly, putative addicts were increasingly cast as degenerates, incorrigible psychopaths, or deranged skid row derelicts (in any case, intrinsically defective and beyond hope of therapeutic reform). As the interest in therapeutic reform declined, so too did scientific interest in whether there were social contextual causes of either addiction itself or recovery (Weinberg 2005). By the mid-twentieth century, most people had come to take for granted that addiction is a largely incurable condition from which only very few ever recover.

This pessimistic outlook was dealt several significant scientific blows in the second half of the twentieth century by research that empirically demonstrated the ubiquity of controlled drug use and outright recovery from addictions that was observed to occur with changes in the life circumstances or social contexts within which former addicts came to live (Heyman 2009). In 1962, Charles Winick (1962) published his bombshell demonstration that most of those who engage in patterns of addictive drug use eventually, to use his own words, "mature out" of these patterns of use naturally as they grow older and more deeply invested in their work, families, and other adult roles. Later, Lee Robins (1993) showed that only very few of those returning Vietnam veterans who had become addicted to heroin in Vietnam resumed their addictions once they came home from the war. Bruce Alexander's (2008, 193–95) "rat park" studies and Norman Zinberg's (1984) work on drug, set, and setting demonstrate that both rodents and humans, respectively, respond and habituate to drug ingestion very differently, depending on the social contexts of ingestion. Waldorf, Reinarman, and Murphy (1991, 10) note that their research subjects who possessed what they called a "stake in conventional life" were both much less likely to fall into self-destructive patterns of drug use and, if in fact they did fall into addiction, much more likely to pull themselves out. This suggested, as does the bulk of epidemiological research, that it is often social rather than genetic or neurological disadvantages that best predict who is most likely to succumb to addictive drug use and who is least likely to recover from it.

Rather than being reducible to the overwhelming chemical allure of drugs or relatively fixed personal characteristics like our genes or "psychopathy," this research suggests that by changing people's social circumstances we may very well be able to change their behavior in ways conducive to their own and society's better flourishing. However, largely due to the enduring legacy of liberalism in both addiction science and popular culture more generally, we do not yet have an approach to linking addictive behavior with social context that does not end up casting that behavior as just a harmful predilection to prioritize immediate self-gratification. But, if indeed addictive behavior is no more than this, in what sense can it be argued to provide adequate grounds for compassion and therapy as opposed to mere disincentives or punishment?

The Brain Disease Paradigm and the Ecology of Addiction

For the most part, disease theorists confine themselves to laboratory science and give at best peripheral attention to social contextual influences on addiction. To the extent they do attend to such factors, they are overwhelmingly cast in Pavlovian terms as "cues" or "secondary reinforcers." According to this argument, drug users come to associate arbitrary elements of the environments within which drug use takes place with the experience of intoxication. These arbitrary elements of the environment thereby come to cue cravings for drugs, which, by virtue of their invariably rewarding biochemical effects in the brain, are understood as "primary reinforcers." This way of modeling environmental factors completely misses the now indisputable fact that the rewards attendant to drug use are not foregone neurological conclusions but are themselves socially, culturally, and personally variable in the extreme.[1]

Moreover, though primary and secondary reinforcers may be relatively easy to separate into discrete variables in laboratories, it is far more difficult to do so in real-world settings. Drug addicts may very well find drug use compelling primarily because drug-using situations are found compelling. Parties, music, and friends, to name only a few putative cues, can be powerful primary reinforcers for drug use as well as cues that trigger a desire for a drug's putatively "intrinsic" biochemical effects. Again, we must reckon not only with the distinctive chemical composition of a drug but also with the social and cultural contexts that give specific meaning to drug use and that are often important sources of people's psycho-emotional orientations to use.

Another difficulty attendant to this theoretical approach is its rather rigid distinction between operant and classical conditioning (M. Lewis 2018). Research has repeatedly shown that stimuli often, perhaps always, acquire their distinctive character as behavioral cues due to the trajectory of practical action under which they are encountered. For example, a cigarette in the hand of a friend may cue a response very different from that cued by a cigarette in the hand of a chef who is making one's meal. In the first case, one's practical trajectory may entail fostering solidarity with a friend. In the second case, one's practical trajectory might entail ensuring they are served an untainted meal and the character of the cigarette as cue will be likewise shaped accordingly. The same ostensible stimulus (i.e., the cigarette) may cue two very different responses. In light of this plasticity, we are well advised not to draw so fine a line between operant and classical conditioning. Courses of human behavior and the cues that constitute our behavioral environments are far more interdependent and dynamic than many brain disease theorists have been prepared to acknowledge.

Above and beyond the challenges of providing for the social contextual variability of drug effects neurologically, it must also be noted that current brain disease theories of addiction speak largely to the hypothesis that heavy drug use increases the propensity of drug users to pursue further drug use rather than addressing the loss of self-control as such. For those of us interested in addiction per se, it is important to note the conspicuous reticence of these theorists to explicitly develop their implicit views of exactly what addicts lose when they lose their self-control. If the loss of self-control is the defining criterion of addiction, as most leaders in the field now readily acknowledge, then it is indispensable that addiction science provide clear concepts of what selves actually are, such that we find them capable of moving into and out of control of human actions in the first place. It is only then that we will learn how addictions might come to attenuate the causal relationship between selves and their actions. To date, disease theorists have remained conspicuously quiet as to the empirical nature of selves and the manner in which drugs might come to undermine them.[2]

Finally, because they tend to treat addiction as essentially an extreme and harmful tendency to prioritize immediate self-gratification, brain disease theorists also tend to encourage images of the addict as inherently impulsive, hedonistic, short-sighted, undisciplined, self-centered, and incapable of deferring gratification—images decidedly inconsistent with the therapeutic treatment of addicts as innocent victims of a disease over which they have no control. So quite contrary to the professed intentions of disease theorists to mitigate the moral blaming of addicts and to defend a medicalized or therapeutic approach to the management of addiction, their theories often actually encourage us to blame the victims of addiction for their fates. In contrast to those who frame addiction as essentially a lust for immediate self-gratification, I would insist addicts literally *use* drugs instrumentally in ways that are always personally meaningful to them (see also Müller and Schumann 2011). And this meaningful use of drugs is always embedded in and at least to some extent practically responsive to socially structured contexts of action.

Choice Theory and the Ecology of Addiction

As was noted in chapter 2, choice theory began to take off in earnest in the fields of economics, sociology, and social psychology, among others, beginning in the 1980s. Choice theorists have been dedicated to showing that putative addictions do not normally resemble anything close to the level of compulsion suggested by disease theorists (Becker and Murphy 1988; Heather and Segal 2017; Heyman 2009; Levy 2013; M. Lewis 2015; Satel and Lilienfeld 2013). Despite holding that addiction is incentive sensitive, most choice theorists have abandoned the effort to explain addiction with orthodox rational choice theory. For example, George Ainslie (1992) and others have influentially argued that addicts are prone not only to prefer present to future rewards but also to hyperbolically discount the prospects of future costs and benefits. In other words, the greater the expectation of immediate reward and the greater the expected intensity of that reward, the more we become vulnerable to temptations to abandon our longer-term plans and preferences. Hyperbolic discounting, though, is not a form of deliberation confined to addicts. It is a widely shared tendency we all exhibit whether we are addicts or not. Hence, by closing the distance between addiction and generic features of human choice making, choice theorists tend toward a normalization of addictive reasoning and volition. This makes it difficult to see why or how addiction should warrant suspension of our default practices of holding ourselves and one another ethically accountable for our actions in favor of a more therapeutic, sympathetic, and exculpatory stance.

Contra choice theory, therapeutic work does not in the first instance require theories that serve only to plausibly explain or justify addicted behavior; it specifically requires theories that allow these behaviors to be, at least partially, ethically disowned. It is only by plausibly distinguishing addicts' free agency, their self-control, from the effects of their addictions that people might be simultaneously understood as amenable to therapeutic empowerment or emancipation from their addictions and somehow also afflicted by an addiction that justifies and demands such a therapeutic engagement in the first place. Furthermore, those struggling to overcome addictions require theories that go beyond merely providing credible justification for absolution or the disowning of past misdeeds. As all who have sought to care for addicts know, recovery is an ongoing exercise of learning to anticipate and prevent the rekindling of people's addictions, and it requires theories that not only facilitate but actually warrant such projects as well.

Choice theorists have made little, if any, headway in this regard. The philosopher Hanna Pickard (2017), for example, offers the enticing possibility of holding addicts responsible for overcoming their addictions but not blaming them for their addictions. But this turns out to be a distinction not between addicts' responsible free agency (which it is the work of therapy to empower) and the agency of their addictions (which might be suppressed and blamed for anticipated relapses). It is a distinction between what she calls "detached" and "affective" blame.[3] Detached blame is retained by Pickard as a basis for both demanding behavioral change and negatively sanctioning problematic behavior. We must renounce only affectively infused spite in response to what Pickard calls the addicts' "disorders of agency." Conspicuously missing from her account are (1) a warrant for the claim that addicts are emancipated rather than merely domesticated by the changes "therapeutically" imposed on them through negative sanctioning and (2) a warrant for viewing addicted choices as somehow "disordered" rather than just blameworthy—that is, a warrant for therapy over criminal corrections or civil retribution. The criminal justice system certainly blames criminals and is not primarily concerned with therapeutically caring for them. But it does nonetheless seek to appear dispassionate in its dispensation of justice—or, in Pickard's language, to favor "detached" over "affective" blame, just deserts over lynch mobs.

Similarly, while vigorously and masterfully critiquing brain disease models for mistaking neurological markers of normal learning as markers of pathological brain damage, the neurologist Marc Lewis (2017c, 35) repeatedly departs from his addiction-reflects-normal-rather-than-pathological-learning-processes thesis into statements that addictive learning neurologically distorts cognitive functioning. This usage of the negatively value-laden term *distort*, with its implications of disfigurement and perversion, is plainly driven by a desire to provide warrant for therapeutic as opposed to punitive interventions. But Lewis offers no explanation for why addiction should be understood as a "distortion" of normal learning. Indeed, he routinely equates the neurology of negatively valued drug addictions with positively valued preoccupations with things like romantic relationships, sports, and summer holidays (M. Lewis 2015, 2017a, 2018).

In sum, addiction science and policy remain to this day largely torn between, on the one hand, the Scylla of a biomechanical reductionism that cannot adequately provide for the social contextual variability of the incentives and disincentives people find for drug use nor for the addict's putative loss of self-control, and, on the other hand, the Charybdis of a liberal voluntarism that makes distinguishing self-control from the pursuit of what we desire axiomatically impossible and hence conceptualizing the idea of enslavement to one's desires—that is, addiction—equally impossible. In both cases, addiction is cast simply as a persistent lust for immediate self-gratification. And in both cases, little, if any, scientific warrant is provided for distinguishing the self-governed pursuit of happiness from the loss of self-control. Because addicts' loss of self-control is so widely presumed to be the sole warrant for a therapeutic rather than punitive orientation to intervention, this is a rather consequential limitation.

Foucault on Practices of Freedom

Contrary to both biomechanical approaches and the reified voluntarism of a generic liberal subject, Michel Foucault insisted that freedom and ethics take their characteristic forms as diverse, contextually embedded products of the specific constellations of power relations within which they emerge and are sustained. Opposing the apostles of unfreedom, Foucault (1987, 114) demanded we take seriously the workings of personal responsibility and discretion exercised through what he sometimes called "practices of freedom." To those who posit a generic self-governing, largely rational liberal subject as an axiomatic historical constant, Foucault maintained that the reality of freedom cannot be adequately specified either in opposition to determinism or without reference to the historically and culturally specific horizons of possibility articulated in and through power relations. In an important further development of this insight, Nikolas Rose, for example, has long been at the forefront of a group of scholars focused on the Foucauldian concept of "governmentality," or the conduct of conduct, by which various sorts of power/ knowledge regimes are given expression not through violence or coercion but through the very operations of freedom itself (Burchell, Gordon, and Miller 1991; Reith 2004; Rose 1990; Rose, O'Malley, and Valverde 2006).

This group has produced an impressive collection of studies that look at governmentality as it occurs through disciplinary programs, including, notably, what Rose has called the "psy" disciplines, such as psychiatry, but also a number of other administrative disciplines, including economics, politics, and indeed Alcoholics Anonymous. These studies persuasively demonstrate just how, through the powerful operation of liberal and neoliberal institutions, people are variously "obliged to be free in certain ways" (Rose, O'Malley, and Valverde 2006, 89) and obliged to conceive of their own freedom in the terms and techniques furnished by different disciplinary matrices. Liberal forms of freedom are shown to be actualized less through resistance to these regimes than through people's participation in them.

However, by so closely yoking their studies of specific practices of freedom to institutionalized forms of disciplinary expertise, these scholars make it rather difficult to understand what, if any, differences might be drawn between an acquiescence to domination and freedom itself. Moreover, they are unclear as to the ontological status of the media on which disciplinary technologies are exercised and the ethical ramifications thereof. As Foucauldians, they can't easily argue that these media consist of biological bodies, as biology is also understood as a historically and culturally specific disciplinary technology itself. The same goes for psychological minds. But despite this ambiguity, there nonetheless remains a consistent implication in this literature that whatever else these media may be, they are always already human, self-governing, and ethically accountable subjects. Though sometimes professing affinities between their own approach and what they call the "antihumanist stance" of Actor Network Theory (Rose, O'Malley, and Valverde 2006, 93), their interest in nonhuman agency has been confined to such matters as prison cells and has not been applied to understanding the specifically intrapersonal forces that may occasionally vex our freedom. As will be shown, this glossing of that which is interior to us as persons but exterior to the free subjectivity of our selves rather limits the potential of this research tradition in certain important ways.[4]

This cannot be quite so easily said of Foucault himself. While arguing that "power exists only over free subjects, and only insofar as they are 'free'" (Foucault 1983, 221), Foucault explicitly contrasted this form of effectuality from the kinds of control that are exercised over things—that is, unfree nonsubjects (Foucault 1983). Immediately following the passage just quoted, Foucault (1983, 221) goes on to write, "By this we mean individual or collective subjects who are faced with a field of possibilities in which several ways of behaving, several reactions, and diverse comportments may be realized. Where the determining factors saturate the whole there is no relationship of power; slavery is not a power relationship when man is in chains. (In this case it is a question of a physical relationship of constraint.)"[5] And most importantly for my argument here, Foucault wrote that while ethical practices are only possible for free subjects rather than slaves or nonsubjects such as prison cells or addictions, conversely, practices of freedom are intrinsically ethical practices.[6]

Of course, Foucault was well aware of the fact that establishing whether a relationship is one of power over free subjects or one of brute determinism often requires a subtle hermeneutics. But there can be no disputing that Foucault provided explicitly for an ethical exterior to the power dynamics that govern relationships between free subjects and those subjects with themselves. To my knowledge, though, he himself never explored this matter in any detail. More specifically, he did not provide for the practical dynamics that produce, nor the resulting ontological status of, those elements of our being, such as addictions, that we dissociate from free will or self-control. Given his deep appreciation for the historicity, contingency, and lability of social life (or to use his own word, its microphysics), it is safe to assume Foucault would have been sensitive to the multiplicity of patterns by which boundaries are drawn between power dynamics and their ethical exteriors. But while Foucauldian insights are immensely conducive to highlighting and examining these patterns, they are not sufficient. We must more closely consider than did Foucault the processes through which particular people evaluate their own and one another's self-identification with, as well as alienation from, their thoughts, feelings, and behaviors.

The Ecology of Addiction, the Divided Habitus, and Self-Actualization

While both brain disease and choice theorists of addiction tend overwhelmingly to assume a more or less unified human subject possessed of habits largely integrated through cost-benefit analysis, research in neurology, psychology, and sociology is beginning to more fully appreciate the pervasive reality of subjective fragmentation and disunity. As noted in chapter 2, Marc Lewis, for example, has argued that habit learning originates in specific settings but that eventually, because brains tend to conserve structure and resources, habits, or acquired "synaptic networks," often converge and become mutually reinforcing. However, he notes, these processes need not converge on a wholly unified subject, or fully integrated hub, for all experience, deliberation, and volition. Instead, "alternative synaptic networks can compete with each other ... this is the case when addiction arises in development, but also when it dissipates, replaced by the desire for and belief in alternative outcomes" (M. Lewis 2017b, 182).

Lewis's distinctive emphasis of neuroplasticity, the setting-specific foundations of habit acquisition, and the possible disunity of our synaptic networks opens an unprecedented path toward what I have here called an ecological understanding of addiction. While he acknowledges a deep intellectual debt to Kent Berridge (2000), who has argued that some substances and/or experiences are intrinsically desirable given the neurological hardwiring of our brains, Lewis never himself explicitly adopts this view and is, as noted, much more likely to highlight neuroplasticity and neurodiversity than hardwired universal dispositions. Unlike most neurologists, then, his work is consistent with the fact that not all people find drug-induced experiences rewarding. It is also consistent with the fact that particular people may find these experiences rewarding under some circumstances and wholly detest them under other circumstances. Lewis's neurological insights in this regard strongly support a view of the body as host to diverse and perhaps conflicting desiring subjectivities. However, though he notes that our habits emerge, develop, and are sustained with respect to specific settings of practical action, he has not pursued this line of inquiry in any significant depth.

We may, however, look to the eminent French sociologist Pierre Bourdieu (1990) for a much more fully articulated approach to the relationship between habit and environmental settings. Bourdieu argued that most of our behavior is not adjusted to our environments consciously or deliberatively but habitually. By participating in and experiencing these environments, we acquire what he called a *habitus*, an implicit, unreflective "feel for the game" or practical sense of what is required to cope in these environments. Likewise, our embodied experience of the various elements that make up these environments is also understood ecologically, or with respect to the practical activities within which those elements emerge as meaningful and practically relevant to us. This approach allows us to much more effectively theorize the sociogenic or environmental influences on drug use, drug experiences, and addiction. It does so by allowing us to avoid the mistakes of treating them either as mere Pavlovian side effects of acontextual neurological processes or as products of self-governed cost-benefit analyses.

A caveat is now in order. Because he was primarily concerned with explaining how people are often unwittingly complicit in preventing their own social mobility, Bourdieu tended to write of a more or less *unified* habitus adjusted for better or for worse to the *general* positions we are normally compelled to occupy in the social world. That said, very good reasons can be found both in Bourdieu's own work and elsewhere to suggest the possibility of a more divided or pluralized habitus. For example, Bourdieu's protégé, Loïc Wacquant (2016, 68–69), writes,

> Habitus is not necessarily coherent and unified. Rather, it displays varying degrees of integration and tension, depending on the character and compatibility of the social situations that fashioned it over time. A sequence of congruent institutions and stable microcosms will tend to fashion a cohesive habitus whose successive layers reinforce one another and work in unison. Dissimilar organizations anchored by divergent values or entropic universes, by contrast, cultivate unstable systems of dispositions divided against themselves and wont to generate irregular and inconsistent lines of action.

Wacquant's invocation of "unstable systems of dispositions divided against themselves and wont to generate irregular and inconsistent lines of action" will no doubt ring a bell for students of addiction. The fact that these dispositions are understood as acquired but preconscious or habitual is also deeply resonant with what we know empirically about addiction. What may be less well established is the premise that these unstable dispositions are products of clashes pressed on us by the ecological contexts of our lives rather than clashes between short-term and long-term preferences. Pertaining to the warrant and facilitation of therapeutic care for addicts, this approach valuably augments what is now a virtually unrivalled understanding of the instability of addicts' dispositions to act in terms of a temporal contrast between short-term and long-term preferences. Despite their earnest hopes to encourage compassion and therapeutic care, the steadfast focus of most addiction scientists on temporal mechanisms of preference instability, such as incentive sensitization and hyperbolic discounting, too often results in images of addicts as impulsive, hedonistic, and incapable of deferring gratification. Weighed down by images such as these, it is very difficult to counter the ubiquitous tendency both among health care professionals and the wider public to blame addicts for their fates.

While we are all prone to greater and lesser degrees of personal integration depending on the extent to which we have been shaped by what Wacquant calls "dissimilar organizations anchored by divergent values or entropic universes," I would argue that the failure of personal integration can sometimes become so extreme as to precipitate a radical personal and moral divestment from fragments of our habitus that effectively divorces those fragments from our own or our significant others' sense of who we really are—that is, more specifically, our addictions from ourselves as self-discovering, self-actualizing, and self-governing ethical subjects. To put this in Foucauldian terms, a failure of personal integration can sometimes compel us to distinguish fragments of our habitus as addictions and as ethically exterior to the particular practices of freedom that constitute us as particular selves. In sum, then, and for a variety of biological, psychological, and social reasons, we may become sufficiently alienated from certain of our habits that we cease to experience them as genuinely our own and instead feel them as afflictions and in some sense enslaving.

This understanding of the environmental influences on addiction also illuminates better than does received addiction science why and how interventions like twelve-step groups and therapeutic communities have been so comparatively attractive to those seeking help with their addictions and to those predisposed to provide such help. In contrast to other forms of therapeutic care, these kinds of interventions seek to emphasize the provision of immersive ecological alternatives to the spaces within which people's addictions were forged and within which they might continue to be rekindled. They are, in other words, comparatively better keyed to the linkage of our habits to the various ecological spaces within which they are acquired and sustained and within which we also evaluate their compatibility with our specific projects of self-discovery and ongoing self-actualization.

POSTHUMANISM, ADDICTION,
AND THE LOSS OF SELF CONTROL
Reflections on the Missing Core
in Addiction Science

There is a curious void at the center of addiction science. Despite widespread acknowledgment that the core criterion of addiction is the loss of self-control (H. Levine 1978; O'Brien, Volkow, and Li 2006; Reinarman 2005; Valverde 1998; West 2006), nowhere has anyone fully succeeded in scientifically distinguishing controlled drug use from the loss of self-control. Whereas the social sciences have tended to construe addiction as either deviant but nonetheless self-governed behavior or discourses thereof, the biomedical sciences have failed even to adequately specify, let alone empirically analyze, how we might distinguish self-governed from addicted behavior. This oversight stems from the overwhelming tendency to conceptualize human biology and human social life dichotomously as two, and only two, wholly discrete and independently integrated ontological domains. While mainstream addiction science allows for research that combines categories from each side of the boundary between "the social" and "the biological," it is largely resistant to considering this boundary as itself diversely drawn, provisional, and in flux. Because posthumanism has been precisely concerned with problematizing this understanding of the relationship between "the social" and its ontological others (e.g., "the natural," "the biological," "the mental," "the metaphysical") and insists that particular configurations of the social and its ontological others are intrinsically mediated through one another, it offers an immensely valuable opportunity to overcome the strange pandemic disability one finds throughout addiction science to account for its own core phenomenon.

In the first section of this chapter, I demonstrate that neither the biomedical nor the social sciences have ever managed to adequately link drug use with a loss of self-control. I then show how this limitation can be very easily overcome by the adoption of a posthumanist perspective on self-control and the various afflictions, including addiction, to which it is regarded heir. This argument provides occasion to acquaint readers with posthumanist scholarship concerning a spectrum of relevant topics, including the human body, disease, drug use, and therapeutic intervention and to show how these lines of investigation can be combined to provide an innovative, theoretically robust, and practically valuable method for advancing the scientific study of addiction specifically as a loss of self-control. The chapter concludes with a discussion of two of the more important ramifications that follow from the adoption of the proposed posthumanist approach to the study of addiction for drug policy studies. The first is a less generic and more nuanced regard for the particular constellations of challenges faced by specific policymakers, service providers, and service users, not least of which is the various combination of factors that can influence the phenomenology of addiction as affliction. Second, precisely because it enhances our appreciation of the phenomenology of addiction as affliction, the proposed posthumanist orientation to addiction also provides for an empirically richer and more nuanced consideration of the ethics of intervention. Scholarly debate on the ethics of intervention has suffered from a too starkly dichotomous characterization of drug use as either a freely exercised prerogative or a symptom of biological pathology. Posthumanism helps us more exactly appreciate the continuum between freedom and affliction as well as the full range of empirical factors that influence how drug-related behavior is specifically located on this continuum in any given instance.

Where in Addiction Science Is the Loss of Self-Control?
A Brief History of Biomedical Approaches to Addiction

A few early modern authorities dabbled with the idea that chronic inebriety may reflect a disease (H. Levine 1978; Porter 1985), but sustained biomedical interest did not emerge until the middle of the nineteenth century.

By the late nineteenth century, there was a fairly well established two-tiered medical understanding of addiction (Courtwright 2001). Those who could afford private care were ordinarily diagnosed with the so-called disease of neurasthenia, literally nervous exhaustion, and prescribed temporary respite from the complex and emotionally taxing demands of modern life. Those who could not afford to pay were consigned to state-sponsored institutions also staffed by medical doctors but designed to manage the more pessimistic diagnosis of degeneracy. Degeneracy followed either from a hereditary predisposition or a dissolute life, and while it could be prevented, few medical men thought it could be reversed. Rather than seeking to return the patient to a former state of nonaddiction, the medical treatment of degeneracy was focused more on limiting the havoc that degenerate addicts might wreak on their wider communities.

In these early days, reigning theories still reflected the influences of humoral medicine in prioritizing attention to moderate habits and self-regulation over anatomical structure and physiological function. And while it would be unfair to blithely reduce nineteenth-century addiction medicine to no more than dressed-up social prejudices, it was undeniably more deeply informed by the perceived character of the patient than the perceived character of their putative disease (Baumohl and Room 1987; Courtwright 2001). In short, insofar as addiction medicine had not yet fully distinguished medical pathology from the social marginality it was meant to explain, it had as yet no clear separation between what a Foucauldian might call the biomedical and the sociocultural gaze. Nor, more specifically, did it provide any way of medically linking drug use with a loss of self-control. Neurasthenia cast addiction as a form of fatigue, not biological dysfunction, and likewise, degeneracy yielded an understanding of addiction as atavism, not affliction. Neither could empirically distinguish self-control from its loss because in neither case was anything other than the self of the supposed addict implicated as a proximal cause of his or her behavior.

As the nineteenth century came to a close, addiction medicine entered a protracted period of doldrums. Theories of degeneracy and neurasthenia were eventually dismissed by a new generation of medical scientists, and the pall of prohibitionist sentiment and then legislation both minimized the availability of funding for addiction research and dissuaded most medical professionals from entering the field. Those who did occupied two camps. The first embraced psychodynamic theories that retained a view of addicts as intrinsically inferior beings (Acker 2002). The second focused on physiological withdrawal, arguing that addiction did not belie underlying deficits such as degeneracy or psychopathy but was a normal physiological response to which anyone might succumb (Campbell 2007). Because they seemed to legitimate medical maintenance of addicts' drug supply, physiological withdrawal-based theories did not enjoy much approval among policymakers committed to prohibition but did slowly gain sway in the medical community as psychodynamic psychiatry fell from favor. Physiological withdrawal symptoms appeared to provide a specific, universally applicable, biomedically identifiable marker by which addicts might be categorically distinguished from nonaddicts. They thereby introduced an apparent path to scientific respectability insofar as the etiology and identity of addiction could now be categorically specified in strictly biomedical terms. Those substances that produce physiological withdrawal symptoms were classed as genuinely addictive. Those that did not were categorically denied that status. However, once again, addiction science had plainly failed to link drug use with a loss of self-control. Demonstrating that a substance causes withdrawal symptoms does not indicate how these symptoms, in turn, cause a loss of self-control rather than just a change and narrowing of personal priorities.[1] Indeed, using drugs to stave off the pains of withdrawal could be seen to exhibit a perfectly reasonable cost-benefit analysis.

Other, better-noticed anomalies also began to accumulate. One can perfectly understand how someone might remain in a perpetual cycle of withdrawal symptom avoidance for as long as withdrawal symptoms actually loom. But why is it, some asked, that the many medications that ease or altogether eliminate physiological withdrawal symptoms have had such a dismal record of getting people permanently off drugs? Perhaps even more perplexing, why are those who have actually suffered the ravages of cold turkey not uniformly chastened by this experience? One would think that such a profoundly nasty ordeal might discourage people from returning to the use of drugs that cause physical dependency. But, too often, it does no such thing. Conversely, why do so many people who become physiologically dependent seem to have so few, if any, qualms about stopping? Finally, it has grown progressively more difficult to argue that only gross physiological withdrawal symptoms cause addiction.[2] Drugs such as crack cocaine or nicotine and activities such as sex, gambling, and eating—none of which produce such symptoms—appear capable of inducing behavioral patterns every bit as damaging as those induced by alcohol and opiates. It is in no small part due to this accumulation of anomalies that interest turned to our most recent paradigm in biomedical addiction science (Leshner 1997, 46), what the historian David Courtwright (2010) dubbed the "NIDA Brain Disease Paradigm."

The brain disease paradigm is first and foremost anchored in the priority given to basic science (Campbell 2010; Vrecko 2010). This has largely meant confining research to basic biology conceived as a primordial, discrete, and independently integrated ontological domain. Brain disease scientists argue that people ingest chemicals such as heroin, cocaine, alcohol, or nicotine because they biologically cause euphoria by promoting the release of neurotransmitters, preventing their reuptake, or mimicking their effects (Koob 2006). But what of addiction? Many studies have noted that after prolonged use the positive effects of drug use are often eclipsed by the negative (Koob et al. 1989). Some heavy users even report that they continue to relapse despite the fact that drugs have long since ceased to give them any satisfaction (Lindesmith 1968). How does the brain disease paradigm account for these seemingly anomalous findings? It does so by suggesting that prolonged drug use induces neurological adaptations that both reduce users' sensitivity to alternative sources of reward and increase sensitivity to the anticipated rewards of drug use. While these adaptations do not produce gross withdrawal symptoms upon cessation of use, they do render people considerably more vulnerable than they might otherwise be to relapse.

How does this model account for addicts' putative loss of self-control? First, according to incentive sensitization theory, the intensity of addicts' desire for drugs is neurologically disjoined from the degree to which they derive pleasure from drug use (Robinson and Berridge 2003). Hence, their felt desire for drugs is apparently unjustified by the degree of benefit that users believe they derive from them. This finding has prompted brain disease scientists to cast this desire as pathological by virtue of its inconsistency with conventional understandings of rational choice. *But conflating the perception of self-control with an abstract model of rational choice is scientifically unsustainable.* Discounting future outcomes in favor of expectations of short-term satisfactions does not logically entail a loss of self-control, nor do people necessarily experience it as such. People often throw caution to the wind with no ensuing inference that they have been pathologically deprived of their self-control. Aside from denigrating their judgment, an adequate scientific account of the loss of self-control must explain why and how people appear to grow estranged from their own behavior enough to warrant the claim that they are genuinely afflicted by something rather than merely exercising limited foresight (Weinberg 2005).

The second way that neurological adaptations to drug use are said to deprive people of their self-control is by compromising brain processes associated with what are often called executive functions (Goldstein and Volkow

2011).[3] These functions are not always clearly delineated in the brain disease literature, but they cover things such as attention, response inhibition, planning, problem solving, working memory, and other such matters pertaining to the evaluation and control of first-order cognitive processes. Like incentive sensitization theory, this research seeks universal neurological measures of self-control. While they may have other scientific merits, such efforts invariably stray rather far from the lived realities and experiences of self-control and its loss among humans outside lab settings. To claim that people uniformly equate their own or each other's self-control with their capacities for long-term planning, problem solving, and impulse control is patently false. Not only do we deliberately throw caution to the wind on occasion but so too on occasion do we equate our "real selves" with our gut instincts, spontaneous sensibilities, or predilections and indeed equate the kinds of activities associated with "executive function" with alienation from our real selves and authentic self-control (Alasuutari 1992, 160–61; Hochschild 2012; R. Turner 1976). Indeed, precisely because they hope to reestablish people's authentic sense of themselves, many rehabilitation programs place extensive therapeutic emphasis not on learning to executively inhibit spontaneous emotions but on "getting in touch" with them through their free and open expression.

This neuroscientific disregard for the manifold empirical permutations of self-control and the loss thereof stems from a manifest inability or unwillingness to breach the boundaries of brain biology in any but the most ancillary manner. The brain disease of addiction is held to occur wholly within the confines of an evolutionarily determined organismic system that all members of our species share more or less in common. Yes, this system interacts with the environment in which it must survive but it does so in a manner preprogrammed by the legacy of its evolution and largely fixed by genetic inheritance. While conditioning may *arbitrarily* link environmental cues with our experience of substances and/or activities deemed intrinsically addictive, it poses no prospect of fundamental divergences between the neurological characteristics of either sufferers or their brain diseases themselves. Instead, conditioning yields only secondary elaborations precisely analogous to the more general relationship neuroscientists draw between the singularity and determinacy of our biological nature as a species and the diversity and impermanence of the cultures we inhabit. In any event, both brain function and dysfunction are understood as mechanically caused by a combination of biological and ecological determinants and hence seemingly nondiscretionary *whether addicted or not*. This mindset will no doubt continue to yield scientific dividends in a variety of ways. But because it does not speak to the physiology underlying the diverse empirical permutations of freedom or self-control in the first place, it cannot yield a scientifically valid grasp of the nuanced phenomenology of being estranged from one's own behavior—that is, losing self-control—nor the jointly intrapersonal, interpersonal, and social structural dynamics that render that estrangement so real for people.

A Brief History of Social Scientific Approaches to Addiction

Let me now allay any concern that this chapter is a one-sided critique of neuroscience. When it comes to grasping the nature and causes of the loss of self-control, social scientific studies have fared no better. In the interest of brevity, I will first quickly dispense, for now, with those approaches that don't seek to explain the loss of self-control in the first place. Rational choice theories argue that any behavior held to exhibit a loss of self-control is in fact entirely self-governed and even, if obscurely, rational (Ainslie 1992; Becker and Murphy 1988; Davies 1992; Orphanides and Zervos 1995). Likewise, much social scientific research looks not at the loss of self-control per se but at the ways in which discourses of addiction have figured in various sociocultural contexts (Alasuutari 1992; Duster 1970; Fraser, Moore, and Keane 2014; Keane 2002; H. Levine 1978; Reinarman 2005; Room 1985; Valverde 1998; Weinberg 2005). As illuminating and important as it is, this literature tends to either reject the claim that people really do sometimes lose control of their drug use and/or beg the question of how such a loss of control might be properly understood. By extant social constructionist lights, we may sometimes suffer from being discursively defined as addicts. But the notion that something other than human subjects, as defining agents, might be the source of suffering has been more difficult to formulate within the constructionist frame.

Since the pioneering work of Alfred Lindesmith (1938b), social scientific research on addiction has given pride of place to social learning and linguistic meaning. As we saw in chapter 1, Lindesmith noted that people who become physiologically dependent on opiates in hospital settings rarely become addicted. He attributed this to their ignorance of the source of their withdrawal distress. Street addicts, on the other hand, generally do know the source of their withdrawal symptoms and how to alleviate them with drug use. Lindesmith argued that, by learning to use drugs to alleviate withdrawal, mere drug users are transformed into genuine drug addicts. Fundamental to his theory was the linguistic meaning people learned to attribute to drugs and their physiological effects. Hence, as we've noted, Lindesmith's theory of addiction relies intrinsically on a division of human perception into (1) brute sensations caused by the body's mechanical response to its physical condition (e.g., withdrawal symptoms) and (2) the mind's active, discretionary, deliberate, and linguistic interpretation of those sensations. This voluntaristic social psychology blocked Lindesmith from coherently theorizing addiction as a loss of self-control or as something suffered rather than chosen. Later social scientific accounts of addiction have also failed to do so.

Seeking wholly social structural explanations, mid-twentieth-century functionalists shared in common a departure from Lindesmith's presumption of a necessary physiological component to addiction. But also as we saw in chapter 1, in so departing, these theories slipped from any pretense of analyzing addiction as a loss of self-control and into analyses of merely deviant drug use (Cloward and Ohlin 1960; Merton 1938). Some functionalists did try to theorize the social psychological dynamics of addiction. The best known of such efforts was "normative ambivalence theory," which argues that drug problems ensue when people are confronted with competing normative orientations to drug use. Deprived of a consistent normative code, people oscillate between approval and disapproval of a given pattern of drug use. But normative ambivalence theory says little if anything of how, when, and why norms come into conflict or, more specifically, why or how normative conflict produces involuntary behavior. Functionalists were not alone in proffering normative ambivalence theories of addiction. Symbolic interactionist Marsh Ray (1961, 140), for example, concludes his classic study of the cycle of abstinence and relapse as follows: "Socially disjunctive experiences bring about a questioning of the value of an abstainer identity and promote reflections in which addict and non-addict identities are compared. The abstainer's realignment of his values with those of the world of addiction results in the redefinition of self as an addict and has as a consequence the actions necessary to relapse."

Here, Ray construes relapse as the effect of a wholly self-governed cost-benefit comparison of being an addict versus being an abstainer. Another symbolic interactionist, Richard Stephens (1991, 180), writes, "Street addicts are generally, what I would refer to as 'rational actors.' To a large extent, they 'choose' to become street addicts." In line with the symbolic interactionist axiom that selves are the inevitable source of all human deliberation and volition, Norman Denzin (1993) defines addiction as an emotionally troubled form of self-government rather than a loss of self-control. And, more recently, Kahryn Hughes (2007, 674) argued that "practices of addiction are about *being one's self.* That is to say, practices of addiction are integral to the process by which addicts constitute and maintain their identity; thus to stop engaging in these practices means, in effect, to stop being themselves." Hughes (2007) is well aware that her position flatly denies that addiction involves a loss of self-control. However, she appears less aware that her position rules out any distinction between what she calls "practices of addiction" and practices of recreational and/or performance-enhancing drug use by nonaddicts. And though Hughes (2007, 689) denies that addiction is reducible to an empirically baseless myth or discourse, emphasizing that addiction "discourses . . . can be understood as both productive and constrained by corporeal experience," her own equation of addiction with practices of the self is demonstrably immune to such constraint. Because this equation predefines all corporeal experiences of drug effects as forms of embodied self-consciousness (drug use is, after all, always self-governed), Hughes must construe the body exclusively as the self's enabling medium. Hence, by definition, the body cannot yield experiences of drug-related constraint or estrangement of one's self from one's embodied drug habits (Leder 1990; Nettleton, Neale, and Pickering 2011).

Addiction science must never forget that the vast majority of drug users are not addicts nor at significant risk of becoming addicts. People use all manner of drugs usually with little disruption to their ordinary practices of self-government (Duff 2004; Reinarman 2013; Waldorf, Reinarman, and Murphy 1991). Drug use is sometimes also incorporated into extraordinary forms of self-government, from binges to raves to sacred rituals. While they are sometimes harmful, practitioners rarely interpret these practices as involuntary. The many temperance crusaders and drug warriors who over the years have labeled such drug uses as evidence of addiction have largely disregarded users' own reports in the name of a priggish denigration and/or punishment of their lifestyles. In the process, they have forsaken the original definition of the term *addiction*—as enslavement—in favor of definitions more akin to terms such as *strange, disgusting, criminal*, or *immoral*. Oddly enough, social scientists have seemed to follow suit in this respect, albeit inversely, largely dismissing as illegitimate users' own reports of a loss of self-control and converting questions of addiction—that is, questions of whether, why, and how people may experience a loss of self-control—into questions of why people break society's rules or why their societies condemn drug use in the first place. I say oddly because social scientists' disregard for people's reports of addiction doesn't appear to be driven by an analogous priggishness or spite.

Instead, inverse to my argument regarding neuroscience, I want to suggest that social scientists' predilection to construe addiction as voluntary deviance or myth is primarily a function of their entrenched commitments to humanism. Social scientists have long been trained to think in terms of integrated groups and to define their members as integrated individuals—rational, self-governing agents that belong to these groups by virtue of shared traditions, interests, and/or values. Thinking within this frame has helped us learn a great deal (though not without limits) about things such as race, class, and gender relations, social control and social deviance, ideologies and myths. But it has been less fruitful in the study of matters such as ecological sustainability, built environments, or, in the present case, the loss of self-control because these latter topics have seemed uncontainable or unaccountable from within our haloed disciplinary categories and presuppositions. Some argue that analytic, or a priori, conceptual partitions and their attendant inclusions and exclusions are part and parcel of the scientific enterprise (Collins and Yearley 1992, 382). Accordingly, we must simply choose a discipline and squeeze as much explanatory power out of it as possible, while remembering that our theories are never simple "mirrors of nature," to use Richard Rorty's (1979) famous phrase. Hughes (2007, 674) seems to take this view when she writes, "I am rejecting a positivist preoccupation with causality . . . , a clinical search for the 'mechanism' of addiction . . . , and instead pointing towards a re-orientation of concepts of 'addiction,' towards a properly social theoretical object."

She also demonstrates a too seldom seen appreciation of the distance this analytic approach can put between our theories and the details of our research subjects' lives. After highlighting the sociological advantages of framing addiction in terms of identity practices and "purposeful relational configurations," she writes,

> It is important to emphasize that addiction and withdrawal have variously been described as a personal hell by the respondent sample drawn upon in this paper. This immediately highlights a core dilemma of academic writing: that in theorising for the purposes of academic exchange we risk losing contact with precisely that which we wish to encapsulate. Vomiting, shaking, lack of sleep, "rattling like hell," the manifold lived experience, the corporeal array of addiction is effectively erased through the use of a technical lexicon. But equally, by focusing precisely on these corporeal aspects because they are so visible and immediate, and those aspects of addiction which we seek to "treat," we risk also obscuring the profoundly social character of addiction. (Hughes 2007, 674)

Yes, indeed! I have so far argued that it is primarily by virtue of their enduring commitment to a largely mechanistic technical lexicon that the biological sciences of addiction have found it virtually impossible to retain what Hughes here calls "contact" with the distinction, let alone transitions, between self-controlled drug use and addiction. The rigid equation of self-controlled judgment and behavior with abstract models of rational choice and/or executive inhibition and problem solving is as close as these sciences have managed to come to what is the manifestly much more richly layered, textured, and nuanced world of drug-related choices and activities. Conversely, it is primarily by virtue of their enduring commitment to a humanist technical lexicon that the social sciences of addiction have also found it virtually impossible to retain contact with the distinction or transitions between self-controlled drug use and addiction. In our efforts to retain focus on its social aspects, we have all but foreclosed on understanding addiction as anything other than a stigmatizing myth, self-indulgence, or, at best, form of normative ambivalence. Each of these approaches secures a social scientific frame of reference at the expense of understanding addiction as a form of affliction or in any way distinguishable from voluntary drug use.

Posthumanism, Bodies, Selves, and Addictions

The humanist tradition pervades Western thought pertaining to politics, morality, law, and art and is very clearly evident throughout the social scientific research on addiction reviewed in this book. Humanists insist that the irreducible atoms of social life are inevitably human subjects—integrated, deliberative agents possessing interests and cultures that endow their worlds with meaning, value, and distinctive rationalities. Posthumanists worry that this imagery reifies human nature and denies the possibility of progressively reformulating or even modifying what it is to be human (Haraway 1991; Hayles 1999). Contrary to humanists, posthumanists do not treat human nature as intrinsically immutable but as something dynamically and diversely constituted through different configurations of practice within which actors, human or otherwise, mutually shape one another (Knorr-Cetina 1997; Latour 2005; Pickering 1995). Finally, eschewing reification, posthumanists examine situated practical action directly for clues as to how things are realized (literally made real) in any actual case. In what follows, I draw upon a collection of posthumanist thinkers to address three topics central to the scientific study of addiction—human bodies, selves, and addictions (understood specifically in the original meaning of enslavements).

Donna Haraway (1991) pioneered posthumanist research on the human body. Trained as a biologist, she combines an insider's understanding with a discerning critical eye. She has, for example, demonstrated the extent to which biologists have variously adopted and legitimated sexist and racist cultural assumptions and thereby exposed the fallacy of the view that biological research is independent of the cultures within which it is practiced. Her work on such matters as the human immune system and cyborgs (actors composed of both living flesh and manufactured technologies) has catalyzed fundamental rethinking of the boundaries of human biological systems and of our humanity more generally. Haraway's contributions demonstrate that biologists are a diverse lot, just as ensconced within the contingencies of history and just as capable of being surprised by the complex workings of our corporeality as anyone else. For Haraway, "the biological" and "the social" are not two monolithic and independent ontological domains but a diverse collection of heterogeneous, sociohistorically dynamic, and often interdependent fields of practical action.

For his part, Bruno Latour (2004) has further illuminated the lived realities of embodiment by revealing the body as not only the mechanical medium through which our minds learn but an intrinsically developing and learning faculty in its own right. Drawing upon perfume makers' "odor kits," used to train "noses" to detect progressively subtler aromatic contrasts, he considers how the body itself can "learn to be affected" (Latour 2004, 205). By learning to be affected, Latour suggests that the body is "articulated" in ever more engaged and engaging ways, such as, for example, the honing of more astute, discerning, and indeed insightful olfactory sensibilities. He transcends the subject/object dichotomy by fusing the active learning subject not with biology's mechanistic theories of the body but the lived body of sentient corporeality. Moreover, he also uses the learning effectuated through odor kits to demonstrate the absurd tendency of the subject/object dichotomy to yield questions such as the following:

> *How accurate* is the perception by the nose of the odours registered in the kit? . . . We will thus be tempted to split odours into two: first, odours as they reside in the world—registered by chromatographs and chemical analysis and synthesis . . . —and second, odours as they are sniffed by an unreliable, wavering and limited human apparatus. . . . In the course of this operation, *the interesting body will have disappeared*: either it will be the nature in us, the physiological body, that is, the chemistry of the nose receptors connecting directly with the tertiary structures of the pheromones and other aerosols, or it will be the subjective embodiment, the phenomenological body that will thrive on the

lived-in impression provided by something "more" than chemistry on our nose.... Either we have the world, the science, the things and no subject, or we have the subject and not the world, what things really are. (Latour 2005, 208)

This absurd tendency lies at the root of addiction science and explains its chronic inability to adequately theorize the distinction between controlled drug use and a loss of self-control. It was seen in withdrawal-based theories that could speak in a universal register to the causal effects of drugs on human physiology but not at all to their effects on human action. While it allows brain disease theorists to assert the primacy of the basic (i.e., unlearned) biochemistry of addiction and relegate the sciences of learning to a secondary role, it conspicuously fails to accommodate the indisputable facts that different people respond to drug ingestion differently or that particular people respond differently in different practical contexts (Robins 1993; Zinberg 1984). This variability goes well beyond incentive sensitization, or the dynamics of wanting, to the very question of whether these experiences are liked, or found pleasurable, in the first place and why. In the words of Richard Moran (2002, 211):

It is sometimes said that certain drugs "produce" pleasure, but this is true only in the same sense that either string quartets or ripe cheeses "produce" pleasure. In both cases we can provide the cause without producing the effect, because the person exposed to either the drug or the music doesn't like it, doesn't see what there is to enjoy in it. What was the very form of hazy, druggy pleasure for someone else is for this person merely some unpleasant dizziness and disorientation. Even here, when we speak of drugs "doing" this or that, finding pleasure in the experience is a matter of being inclined to take pleasure in what is given. And the fact that such "know-how" may simply come naturally or spontaneously to the person does not make his engagement any the less active, anymore than it does for ordinary physical skills or habits of inference.

By highlighting that the body is not just an evolutionarily determined mechanical system about which we can learn but, fundamentally, a mutable medium literally articulated through its learning to be affected, Latour goes a considerable distance toward creating a conceptual space within which addiction might be construed as a thoroughly learned pattern of embodied practice. Unlike learning theories of addiction that focus on task-specific habits (like lever pushing in rats), Latour offers a more complex and nuanced orientation to embodied sensibilities closer to the kind Pierre Bourdieu called habitus.[4] It treats sensory perception and evaluative appreciation as mutually implicative and intimately tied to the acquisition of aptitudes for thriving in specific niches. It encourages us to substitute the neurologically reduction-ist understanding of "reward" with a more nuanced and malleable notion of what I call felicity—wherein the pleasurability of drug effects is not a neu-rological fait accompli but derives to a considerable extent from perceptions of a felicitous fit between drug effects and the practical demands of specific situations. Unfortunately, though, Latour (2004) seems to suggest that all ways the body has learned to be affected must inevitably enrich our lives. Clearly, the study of addiction advises a more cautious view. I suggest that by learning to be affected, the body can develop disabling as well as enabling patterns of engagement with the world. Moreover, though he speaks of the multiplicity of environments within which the body learns to be affected, La-tour (2004) does not explicitly address the multiplicity of the body itself—as not just a medium for learning to be affected but a linked set of media for do-ing so. This limits the sensitivity of his model to the potentials for embodied conflicts and/or afflictions such as addiction.

This limitation is also evident in the work of one of the earliest writers to introduce posthumanist insights into the study of drug use and addiction themselves. Taking issue with the liberal philosophical antinomy between the human subject as absolutely free and the body as mechanically deter-mined, Emilie Gomart (2002, 2004) conceptualized drug use and addiction as vehicles for the articulation of human subjectivities rather than inevitably destructive of them. Similar to Latour and Moran, Gomart highlights that taking pleasure in drug use entails our learning to be the kinds of subjects that can do so and is decidedly not an inevitable effect of biochemistry. She describes how despite physiological dependence, the people she studied were often active and tactical users of drugs rather than mere slaves to them. In-deed, even their physiological dependence on methadone is characterized as a "generous constraint" on their actions that allows clinic workers to simul-taneously coerce/seduce drug users into adopting more stable and less risky forms of life. What is conspicuously absent from her studies, though, and what I am seeking to develop in my own work, is an explicit account of why and how addictions might become things that can afflict people, cause them to suffer, and from which we might, on occasion, seek to free them. Hence, unlike Gomart, I do not conceptualize addiction as a universal relation be-tween the generic human body and a psychoactive chemical compound. I have deliberately avoided this because most drug users do not become addicted even if they do become physiologically dependent. Instead, following the lead of my research subjects, I conceptualize addictions as nonhuman agents residing in the bodies of those who are addicted (Weinberg 2005). This conceptualization has required that I go beyond Latour's and Gomart's specifications of human bodies as various types of situationally created singularities and to theorize human bodies as themselves often multiplicities.

Though I will return to Latour's notion of the body as learning to be affected, I must first make clear how such a body can be understood as a form of multiplicity rather than singularity and, perhaps more importantly, how such a body can be understood as subject to harms and afflictions as well as healthy growth and development. In her classic text *The Body Multiple*, Annemarie Mol (2002) highlights how the embodied reality and consequentiality of disease vary depending on the locally organized practices within which disease is observed and engaged. By examining the practical work of clinicians and pathologists on atherosclerosis, Mol found they were dealing with very different things.

> The practices of enacting clinical atherosclerosis and pathological atherosclerosis *exclude* one another. The first requires a patient who complains about pain in his legs. And the second requires a cross section of an artery visible under the microscope. These exigencies are incompatible, at least: they cannot be realized simultaneously. This is not a question of words that prove difficult to translate from one department to the other. Surgeons and pathologists who talk with one another tend to understand each other very well. It is not a question of looking from different perspectives either. Surgeons know how to look through microscopes and pathologists have learned to speak with living patients. The incompatibility is a practical matter. (Mol 2002, 35)

Of course, practitioners can and do abstract their work objects from the details of that work to posit independent things such as cases of atherosclerosis. They thereby link the work objects of clinicians and pathologists as aspects of a singular abstract case. However, Mol notes, this abstraction requires a new kind of practical work that clinicians and pathologists are not always called on to do and the outcomes of which are often uncertain. Clinical findings of atherosclerosis are sometimes confirmed in the pathology lab and vice versa, but not always. Robust clinical findings are sometimes inconsistent with those from the lab. If we attend to the details of medical practice rather than the abstractions of medical knowledge, we discover that practitioners inhabit not a universe—that is, a domain composed of familiar objects that behave together as a system—but a multiverse composed of heterogeneous, unpredictable, and often unfamiliar objects that are not always amenable to being domesticated and made predictable through the creation of knowledge (see also Law and Singleton 2005). Moreover, even if we succeed in securing it, this knowledge is itself inevitably subject to anomalous findings, noise, and revision, if not outright falsification.

Transposed to the field of addiction, Mol's insights shine brightly. In the first instance, they remind us that the realities of addiction, those we seek to understand, are not at all identical to the abstractions proffered by scientists or anyone else to map them. Instead they are to be found in the embodied configurations of local practice within which the specific details of particular people's sense of estrangement from their drug use takes shape.[5] We see that science is sometimes confined rather than empowered by its lexicological commitments. This has been notoriously true in the addiction sciences, where struggles to provide for that thing or things that categorically distinguish addicts from nonaddicts have vexed scientific research almost beyond hope. Examining drug problems in practice reveals a truly breathtaking variety of patterns according to which people use drugs and sometimes develop problems. But by Mol's lights, such multiplicity poses no problem at all. No longer are we concerned with the essence of the abstraction—addiction—that all addicts share in common. Instead, attention is turned to the local details of practice within which people are variously compelled to construe events as evidence of addiction. This is much more likely to reveal not a singular essence of addiction but what the philosopher Ludwig Wittgenstein (1958) called family resemblances among the many ways in which particular people's specific addictions are configured. The attention to local practice should also cure us once and for all of the callous theoretical prejudice that all putative addicts inevitably self-identify with their drug-using practices and never dread or feel tormented or terrified by them.

Modifying Latour's model of the body as learning to be affected by way of Mol's attention to multiplicity, we can say that addictions take form as bodily articulations—that is, as learned embodied sensibilities and felicities that tend to bind us to the worlds within which they are acquired and can be availed (Hughes 2007; Nettleton, Neale, and Pickering 2011). Such binding is not simply a matter of consciously investing in relationships by which drugs and/or the resources necessary to get them can be obtained. It entails the development of embodied tastes and talents for myriad aspects of the worlds in which drug use figures, of tacitly learning literally to *inhabit* these worlds or engage and be engaged by them. As any user will tell you, intoxication is never experienced as the isolated biological effects of drugs in the brain but is inevitably a complex of mutually influential processes wherein drug ingestion combines with other things like feelings of safety or danger, ease or anxiety, food, music, conversation, physical contact, urban landscapes, and myriad others to form fluid gestalts that cannot be experientially disaggregated and that profoundly affect whether and how people experience drug use as pleasurable or not (Duff 2008). Neither felicitous and performance-enhancing nor distressing and performance-debilitating drug use can be adequately understood in artificial isolation from the specific practical and relational contexts within which pleasure and pain, personal ease and dis-ease, or competent and incompetent performance receive their genuine measure.

So how, then, do these Latourian bodily articulations transition between practical felicities and impractical afflictions, between practices of the self and practices of addiction? The body is not an integrated medium through which we learn to be affected but a complex constellation of such media. The assorted articulations of our bodies having learned to be affected will inevitably differ in the extent to which they are enjoyed or esteemed, resented or reviled by ourselves or our significant others. This will largely dictate whether, and the comparative extent to which, we self-identify with our body's different articulations and the comparative extent to which our significant others identify us with some rather than others.[6] For example, my body has learned to be affected by both music and road traffic but I am usually considerably fonder of the former and more likely to self-identify as a lover of music than a lover of traffic. My sons, on the other hand, tend to associate me much more with my ability to drive than with my musical connoisseurship, which in fact they gravely doubt. We also differ with respect to our relative freedom to leave or transform the environments within which particular bodily articulations have developed and are felt necessary. And, inevitably people will also exhibit more and less refined bodily articulations with respect to particular practices and wider and narrower ranges of articulations pertinent to different practices. All these variables combine to determine the extent to which people may (1) be prone to concentrate their energies in few or many different bodily articulations, (2) enjoy or suffer from their engagement in any given form of bodily articulation, and (3) be more or less equipped to discontinue engagement with a given form of bodily articulation. A sense of estrangement or loss of self-control over one's bodily articulations pertaining to drug use emerges when (1) these articulations are perceived to chronically interfere with others from which one derives a greater sense of felicity or self-esteem and (2) one's perceived capacity to discontinue these bodily articulations is somehow compromised, as when, for example, people feel they cannot sleep without sedatives, relax without alcohol, work without amphetamines, or believe in themselves without cocaine.

Robins's (1993) findings of minimal relapse to heroin use among returning Vietnam veterans; Waldorf's (1983) and Biernacki's (1986) findings of a commonly experienced association of recovery from addiction with removal from the types of settings and associates that had constituted one's practical contexts of drug use; and the widely recognized recovery advantage had by addicts with comparatively wider ranges of coping skills and what Waldorf, Reinarman, and Murphy (1991, 10) call a "stake in conventional life" each suggest that drug use is usually a more or less setting-specific form of bodily articulation and that the sense of a loss of self-control is heavily informed not only by the dyadic biological relationship between user and drug but by the wider and more various constellations of practical and relational contexts one has come to inhabit and within which one feels compelled to live. Seen in this light, the status of addiction as a form of dis-ease need not be decided with rigid reference to whether suffering can be decisively linked to dysfunctional biological mechanisms but, more generally, with reference to any number of different patterns of seemingly harmful and intransigent bodily articulation— that is, patterns of bodily articulation with which we cannot, or do not want to, identify ourselves precisely because they appear to afflict or endanger those articulations with which we do self-identify.

What about Policy?

There is at the moment a substantial disconnect between brain disease science and public policy. This is largely because it has yet to yield any significant contributions to either law enforcement or clinical practice (Courtwright 2010). Meanwhile, ascendant social science is far more likely to clash with both law enforcement and clinical approaches to addiction than fruitfully contribute to them. Social scientists are for the most part deeply critical of reigning drugs policy, well aware of their marginality in drug policy debate, and therefore considerably more attentive to their prospects of contributing to debates within the social sciences than to those being waged in the broader public sphere. While I am rather typical in these respects, I do believe that posthumanism offers novel opportunities for closing the distance between social scientific and public policy debate. Due to space constraints, I will raise only two such opportunities.

First, because posthumanism remains closely attentive to the details of situated practice rather than general theory, it is considerably more likely to remain attuned to the range of practical challenges that specific policymakers, service providers, and service users actually face and hence to offer knowledge that is more closely keyed to those challenges. In particular, posthumanism can examine, more seriously than other social scientific approaches, not only the idea that some people really do experience a loss of control over their drug use but also the concrete combinations of intrapersonal, interpersonal, and social structural dynamics that give shape and stability to their addictions and recoveries in situ. In this way, posthumanism represents a form of social constructionism that can remain considerably more loyal to the concerns of our research subjects than others have proven able. This should raise the likelihood that posthumanist insights will succeed where others have failed to pique the interests of service providers and policymakers alike.

Second, posthumanism allows us to much more methodically explore the crucial policy question of whether and when clinical treatment is empowering or oppressive. Whereas brain disease theorists' lack of an adequate concept of self or self-control prevents them from pronouncing at all on whether treatment is empowering or oppressive, the social scientific tendency to view addiction as rational and/or self-governed often yields a blanket construal of all efforts to subdue addictive behavior as necessarily oppressive. The posthumanist approach outlined in this chapter allows an escape from this antinomy between mechanistic neuroscience and humanistic social science by remaining analytically supple enough to provide for the wide range of ways that both drug use and nonuse can either enhance and empower us or distress and disable us in any actual case. In place of the binary opposition between self-control and enslavement to drugs, the proposed posthumanist approach highlights the limits that will inevitably attend any effort to distinguish self-controlled drug use from the loss of self-control in the generic or universalistic terms so much favored by conventional science and evidence-based medicine. It highlights that findings of self-control and affliction are not ordinarily made in accordance with generic diagnostic criteria but on the basis of a much more subtle, holistic, and dynamic regard for the details of particular people's personalities, their patterns of drug use, and the myriad conditions under which they have, are presently, and are anticipated to have to live. It insists that people's regard for these matters is often marked by not only ambiguity and ambivalence but also disagreement and debate. Drug users, their drug-using associates, their friends and families, clinicians, lawyers, and judges, to name only a handful of prospectively relevant actors, often play influential roles in these debates and are more or less influenced by the interventions of one another. This, rather than the intrinsic unreality of addiction, is what explains the equivocalities that can often attend the distinction between self-controlled and uncontrolled drug use even in particular cases. However, in stark contrast to much of the poststructuralist literature (Sedgwick 1993), the proposed approach is not concerned with deconstructing the literary figure of the addict as such but with providing analytic resources with which to describe and explain the composition of selves, bodies, enhancements, and afflictions in particular places and at particular times, incarnate and in all their specificity. These processes are eminently amenable to empirical explanation. It is by means of this provision that I have hoped to contribute to both theory and policy.

An Exchange with John F. Galliher on
Lindesmith's Theory of Addiction

The following exchange was published in *Sociological Theory* 16, no. 2 (1998), on pages 205–8, in response to the author's article "Lindesmith on Addiction: A Critical History of a Classic Theory," which appears as chapter 3 in the present volume. The chapter first appeared, in an earlier version, in *Sociological Theory* 15, no. 2 (1997), on pages 150–61.

"COMMENT ON WEINBERG'S 'LINDESMITH ON ADDICTION'"
John F. Galliher

Minds and Bodies: Staking out the Intellectual Territory

Weinberg's recent study ("Lindesmith on Addiction: A Critical History of a Classic Theory," *Sociological Theory* 15 [1997]: 150–61), financed by the National Institute of Drug Abuse (NIDA), takes up the attack on Lindesmith's theory of addiction, which was for decades an object of scorn by the Federal Bureau of Narcotics and the late Harry J. Anslinger, the bureau's long-time director. Without attributing any particular motives to Weinberg, given what is known about official policy, it is not surprising the NIDA and other U.S. Government agencies encourage and support criticisms of Lindesmith's work. In any case, Weinberg (1997, 151) correctly noted that "Lindesmith made the symbolically mediated interpretations his subjects conferred upon their actions and [physical] experiences the central element of his theory." Weinberg argued that the position of Lindesmith and other symbolic inter-actionists was selected by these sociologists more for tactical than intellectual reasons to compete for professional advantage with other disciplines, espe-cially psychology. The consequent prominence given to symbolic interpreta-tions, Weinberg claims, created a "mind-body dualism [which] is untenable on both epistemological and phenomenological grounds" (150). The problem with Weinberg's assertions is that Lindesmith never claimed this dualism.

Again and again Lindesmith emphasized that people become addicted af-ter experiencing physical withdrawal and learning what it is and how to in-terpret it from their cultural environment. It is misleading to refer to this intimate relationship between physical reactions and human learning as a "dualism."

Of Mice and Men, and Lindesmith

In addition, Weinberg noted that during the 1960s the research findings of behavioral psychologists studying rats demonstrated that rodents could be conditioned to drug use, but "Lindesmith remained extremely resistant to the notion that 'lower animals' can become addicts in the same sense as can human beings" (154). Following the publication of these animal studies Wein-berg reasoned that Lindesmith could no longer argue for the centrality of symbols in addiction. Although Weinberg (159) recognized the significance of "settings and associates" he surprisingly ignored the more variable impact of drugs on the human actor depending on the cultural and symbolic context. Unlike rats, who generally can be conditioned at approximately the same rate, the consequences for the human can be minimal to none as in infants and hospital patients, or overwhelming as in the case of addicts on the street. Ac-cording to Lindesmith, unlike other animals, humans have self-concepts and thus can see themselves as objects. "A drug user does not realize his addiction until he discovers the difficulty of breaking off the habit, and it is this diffi-culty which compels him to accept, however unwillingly and painfully, the idea that he has become a 'dope fiend'" (Alfred R. Lindesmith and Anselm L. Strauss, *Social Psychology*, rev. ed. [New York: Holt, Rinehart and Winston,

1956], 354). Thus, Lindesmith was correct in maintaining a firm distinction between rats and humans.

Lindesmith on Freedom and Constraint

According to Weinberg, adopting the position of symbolic interaction that humans are dynamic beings who are constantly being created and free from psychological determinism placed Lindesmith at odds with his policy position that addicts' "perceptions and actions were beyond their willful capacity to control" (155). Lindesmith "was not able to reconcile his manner of theoretically emphasizing meaning and social learning with his campaign to decriminalize and medicalize addiction" (156). In other words, if people are already free, they do not need to be freed, and moreover, Lindesmith did not describe "learning process through which addicts might progressively lose control over their actions and interpretations" (156). Contrary to this view, Lindesmith argued that it is punitive drug laws that make equally constraining self-conceptions among addicts who have experienced the horrors of withdrawal occasioned by the artificial scarcity produced by legal prohibition. However dynamic in its creation, once the addicted self is created it is a compelling force. Lindesmith sums up the situation as follows: "The principal deleterious effects are psychological in nature and are connected with the tabooed and secret nature of the habit; with the extreme cost of obtaining a supply of drugs at black-market prices; and with resulting changes in self-conception, occupation, and social relationships" (Lindesmith and Strauss 1956, 353). Lindesmith's writing always emphasized that the real horrors of physical withdrawal from drugs were made possible by human self-concepts and magnified many times over by draconian criminal penalties. There is no mind-body dualism here, no confusion of rats and people, nor any false sense of human freedom for American drug addicts.

"PRAXIS AND ADDICTION: A REPLY TO GALLIHER"
Darin Weinberg

Great truth wants to be criticized, not idolized. —FRIEDRICH NIETZSCHE

Galliher suggests my paper is guilty of four failings: (1) it is an "attack" on Alfred Lindesmith that is ideologically consistent with those mounted by Harry Anslinger and the Federal Bureau of Narcotics, (2) it misleadingly casts the "intimate relationship between physical reactions and human learning [in

Lindesmith's theory of addiction] as a [mind-body] dualism," (3) it ignores the "variable impact of drugs on the human actor depending on the cultural and symbolic context," and (4) it erroneously asserts that Lindesmith's commitment to the Blumerian position that "humans are . . . free from psychological determinism" is theoretically irreconcilable with Lindesmith's policy position that addicts' actions and interpretations are beyond their control. Let me rebut each of these claims in turn.

Harry Anslinger was an early and active proponent of a federal war on drugs and his attacks on Lindesmith were based on his commitment to prosecuting drug users as criminals rather than providing addicts with therapy. Nowhere in my paper do I even vaguely imply an endorsement of this policy or the federal war on drugs. As did Lindesmith in his day, I abhor the prosecutorial frenzy embodied in the war on drugs and its transparently repressive, racist, and classist consequences. I favor socially sensitive modalities over strictly medical modalities of addiction treatment and feel that a praxiological understanding of human learning offers sounder theoretical grounding for such modalities than does Lindesmith's exclusively symbolic understanding of human learning. No doubt, Lindesmith's theory of addiction was a watershed achievement in American sociology. By demonstrating the centrality of meaning and social learning to the addiction process, Lindesmith took enormous theoretical strides beyond the biologically and psychologically reductionist theories that had hitherto held the day. Unfortunately, however, Lindesmith's Blumerian social psychology prevented his making conceptually rigorous *sociological* contributions to our understanding of the visceral, or *prereflective and nonsymbolic*, features of drug use, drug-induced experience, and addiction.

Galliher acknowledges that Lindesmith's theory of addiction posits an "intimate relationship between physical reactions and human learning," but, oddly enough, he rejects my assertion that Lindesmith's presumption of such a "relationship" logically requires a categorical distinction *between* brute physical reactions and human learning processes. To argue that Lindesmith never explicitly endorsed a mind-body dualism in the abstract is irrelevant. Lindesmith's theory of addiction is logically incoherent unless one accepts the view that human experience consists in two categorically distinct forms of perception—bodily perception and mental perception. According to this view, bodily perception consists in brute sensations that arise as unmediated outcomes of physical stimuli and are pristinely immune to social influence. Conversely, mental perception consists in the voluntary projection of linguistic categories onto brute sensations and is the sole medium for the meaning, social learning, and practical relevance we find in human experience. This is Lindesmith's (and Blumer's) position, it is a mind-body dualistic account of human perception, and it has been soundly discredited by theorists throughout the human sciences (see my paper for a small sampling of cites).

Galliher's claim that I ignore the "variable impact of drugs on the human actor depending on the cultural and symbolic context" is also plainly mistaken. The crux of my effort was to theoretically strengthen and extend Lindesmith's claim of the importance of meaning and social learning to the addiction process. Nowhere in my paper do I assert, or even imply, that human drug using practices are equivalent to those found in laboratory animals. The point I actually made was that the animal studies proved, contra Lindesmith, that linguistic competence is not a necessary prerequisite to the occurrence of learning processes through which prolonged, self-destructive attachments to the use of drugs take place. In the last section of my paper I provide a praxiological account for the fact that the effects of drug ingestion vary significantly with people's meaningful experience of the settings in which they use drugs, the associates with whom they use drugs, and the practical demands they perceive these settings and associates to entail. I suspect Galliher's misreading of my claims in this respect derive from the common misconception that specifically *cultural* contexts are, by definition, comprised solely of people's symbolic representations of brute phenomena. Lindesmith certainly promoted this view and, alas, some contemporary sociologists continue to do so. In contrast, I suggest the meanings and practical relevances that attach to drugs are not products of *learning to symbolically represent drug-induced physical sensations* but derive directly from the ways people *learn to use drugs as resources in culturally and historically specific fields of practical action*. This is not to argue symbolic interpretations are never influential. Rather, it is to insist that interpretation is ordered by the primordial logic of praxis and to summarily reject the fallacy of brute sensation.

With respect to the issue of freedom and constraint, the historical record unequivocally bears out my claim that Blumer was in fact resolutely committed to a voluntarist understanding of meaningful human action and subjectivity and that Lindesmith never repudiated the Blumerian approach to meaning and social learning. Since Lindesmith always followed Blumer in casting meaningful human action as, by definition, reflective, symbolic, and *self*-determined, he never adequately provided for the possibility of a social learning process through which selves might progressively lose control over their personal actions and interpretations. As an alternative to Blumerian voluntarism, I invoked Bourdieu's notion of habitus as an aid to theorizing how people's propensities toward certain drug experiences and uses, *though socially learned and thoroughly suffused with meaning*, are still often non-symbolic, prediscursive, prereflective, unwitting, and perhaps involuntary. I still regard this a useful fortification and extension of Lindesmith's seminal insights and hence a valuable contribution to sociological theory.

1   As Daniel Breslau (2000, 293) wryly writes, "It is safe to say that no one has ever observed an instance of scientific knowledge constrained by an unknowable and meaningless material world."

CHAPTER 1. SOCIOLOGICAL PERSPECTIVES ON ADDICTION

An earlier version of this chapter appeared in *Sociology Compass* 5, no. 4 (2011): 298–310.

1   References to "drugs" are used in this chapter as a proxy for all putatively addictive substances and/or behaviors, whether or not they actually involve drugs.

2   To be clear, my effort here is not to theoretically define the objective nature of addiction once and for all but to (1) promote a greater terminological precision in empirical sociological research on addiction and (2) examine the idea that addictions, however defined, might sometimes be experienced as sources of human suffering. Those who have sought to understand addiction as a type of affliction or source of suffering have overwhelmingly done so by defining addiction as something that causes a "loss of control," and so it is the sociology of addiction as the loss of control that I am most concerned to explore here. To be sure, a great deal of important sociological research has looked not at the loss of self-control but at how claims regarding the dangers of addiction have figured in campaigns of social control. As vitally important as it is, this largely social constructionist research tends to either completely reject the claim that some people really do sometimes lose control of their use of drugs and/or begs the question of how such a loss of control is best understood sociologically. By extant social constructionist lights, we may sometimes suffer from being defined in one way or another. But the notion that something other than human

subjects, as defining agents, might be the source of suffering has been more difficult to formulate within the social constructionist frame. My hope for this book is to show that this need not be the case.

3 By "gross physiological withdrawal symptoms," I mean symptoms like vomiting, cramping, delirium tremens, runny nose, itchy eyes, and so on, which implicate specific physiological effects of withdrawal. This is in contrast to more psychological effects like anxiety or stress headaches, which are less clearly linked to specific physiological effects of withdrawal.

4 Though informed by symbolic interaction and using a qualitative approach to studying the meaning of drug involvement, Marsh Ray's (1961) influential theory of relapse to heroin addiction is in essence a normative ambivalence theory. Likewise, some learning theories of drug and alcohol problems also exhibit strong affinities with normative ambivalence theories (Akers 1992).

5 Timothy Rouse and Prabha Unnithan (1993) have contrasted responses to alcohol problems in the United States with those in the Soviet Union and found that while, in the United States, responses are largely informed by Protestant ideology, responses in the Soviet Union are informed by what they call a proletarian ethic. Both approaches, however, seem to hinge on efforts to discourage unproductiveness in the political economic system.

6 Of course, different commentators, including addicts themselves, often debate the characteristics of their own and one another's addictions as well as the degree of influence their addictions have over their personal conduct in any given instance. But the fact that the characteristics and relative influence of people's addictions on their activities are intrinsically contestable hardly disqualifies them from being taken seriously as causal agents. Indeed, posthumanist social theory teaches us that it is precisely in this resistance to unequivocal description and decisively unilateral human control that nonhuman agencies are most robustly in evidence.

CHAPTER 2. FREEDOM AND ADDICTION IN FOUR
DISCURSIVE REGISTERS: A COMPARATIVE HISTORICAL
STUDY OF VALUES IN ADDICTION SCIENCE

An earlier version of this chapter appeared in *History of the Human Sciences* 34, nos. 3–4 (2021): 25–48.

1 While these issues have not received much explicit attention in the ethnography of addiction, they have been lucidly analyzed by some in the now burgeoning anthropology of ethics—see especially James Laidlaw's (2014) *The Subject of Virtue: An Anthropology of Ethics and Freedom*. Jarrett Zigon's work (2007, 2011, 2019) contributes to, and draws upon, this literature in analyses of important aspects of addiction and recovery, but it does not address the central issues raised here—the difficulties of informing and warranting therapeutic care for addicts that arise as a consequence of aspiring to value neutrality and universality.

2 Among other accolades, Professor Hyman is a former director of the National Institute of Mental Health (1996–2001), editor of the *Annual Review of Neuroscience,* a fellow of the American Academy of Arts and Sciences, a fellow of the American Association for the Advancement of Science, and a Distinguished Life Fellow of the American Psychiatric Association.

3 One particularly well-known example from the late sixteenth century is the close association William Shakespeare drew between physical disability and moral corruption in *Richard III.*

4 The celebrated Georgian physician George Cheyne wrote in 1725, "The infinitely wise Author of Nature has so contrived *Things,* that the most remarkable rules of preserving Health are moral duties commanded us, so true it is, that Godliness has the promises of this Life, as well as that to come" (quoted in Rosenberg 1992, 54, n. 59). See also Benjamin Rush in 1799: "Christianity when believed, and obeyed . . . is more calculated to produce those effects, than any other religion in the world. Such is the salutary operation of its doctrines, and precepts upon health and life, that if its divine authority rested upon no other argument, this alone would be sufficient to recommend it to our belief" (Runes, 1947, 171).

5 It is worth underlining that in both the early modern Puritan and civic republican discourses, the relevant model for understanding the relationship between freedom and addiction was not free will versus biological determinism but free will versus slavery. Unlike biological determinism, slavery can be understood as a contextually variable form of unfreedom, a matter of degree in the sense that one can be more or less enslaved and one that may grow more and less influential through time. It thus tends to preserve a degree of autonomous (if severely attenuated) personal judgment for the afflicted actor that is not so well preserved in discussions of biological determinism.

6 This formulation draws on Rom Harre's (1987, 42) distinction between the *person* (understood as the "human being as a social individual embodied and publicly identifiable") and the *self* (understood as "that inner unity to which all personal experience [and, I would add, conduct] belongs as attributes of a subject").

7 Hedonic values concern our desires and are those that have traditionally preoccupied utilitarian calculations regarding the rational pursuit of happiness. Eudaemonic values, on the other hand, concern virtue as such. This contrast allows us to distinguish judgments of personal desire from judgments of what it would mean to flourish—what, in other words, is conducive to our personal well-being above and beyond the satisfaction of personal desires or, for that matter, above and beyond our devotion to enshrined ethical principles (see Ryan and Deci 2001; B. Turner 2018).

An earlier version of this chapter appeared in *Sociological Theory* 15, no. 2 (1997): 150–61.

1 I am following Pierre Bourdieu's (1975, 19) usage of the expression "scientific field": "The scientific field is the locus of a competitive struggle, in which the specific issue at stake is the monopoly of scientific authority, defined inseparably as technical capacity and social power, or, to put it another way, the monopoly of scientific competence, in the sense of a particular agent's socially recognized capacity to speak and act legitimately (i.e., in an authorized and authoritative way) in scientific matters."

2 In an analysis of scientific conduct and experience that strikes me as analogous to the analysis of drug use and drug-induced experience I am offering here, Andrew Pickering (1993) describes the process through which physicists adopted the bubble chamber as a resource for the accomplishment of their work. Pickering suggests that physicists would not have adopted the bubble chamber as a practical resource if they had not experienced it as at least potentially conducive to accomplishing the practical projects for which it was engaged. He notes, however, that this claim does not require him to adopt a realist understanding of physical science or the physical world. *Mutatis mutandis*, the same point goes for my analysis of drug use. To claim that people would not likely feel compelled to use a drug if they had not experienced its use as conducive to the accomplishment of particular practical projects does not demand a realist view of the biochemical effects of drugs on human consciousness. The efficacy of the bubble chamber, and of drugs, is experienced by way of, and with respect to, the experiencer's historically and culturally emergent practical activities and not the determinate physical (or neurological) structures of the physical or psychopharmacological essentialist. However, this analytic tack by no means entails rejecting the relevance of biochemical, psychopharmacological, or neurological insights to our understanding of drug-induced experience and addictive drug use. It only calls for a rejection of the proposition that the biochemical changes that occur when certain drugs are introduced into human bodies are themselves the sole producers of specific kinds of experiences, no matter what the praxiological context of drug administration happens to be.

3 Unlike Denzin's (1993) theory of the alcoholic self, the phenomenological perspective I am sketching here suggests one's self is only a possible feature, not a necessary one, within the constellation of thoughts and actions that will be evoked by the perceived demands of a given context of practical action. According to this approach, "the self" is invoked only as it occurs emically, as a percept of the agent, and not etically, as the theoretically defined analytic hub of all lived experience that it is for Denzin. So, in this approach, it is indeed sensible and consistent to speak of someone losing their self in a given course of practical action.

An earlier version of this chapter appeared in *Social Problems* 47, no. 4 (2000):
606–21.

1 The term *ecology* is used here for two reasons. First, it connotes the material-
ity of an environment more than does the term *culture*, which is often held to
refer only to "webs of significance," or symbolic environments (Geertz 1973).
Second, and more importantly, the term *ecology* indicates a reciprocal relation
between agent and environment without presuming the humanity of the agent
in question. Insofar as members of my research settings construed their addictions as disease agents, and not human agents, it is useful to avoid anthro-
pomorphic terms when describing their accounts of the environments within
which their addictions were held to thrive.

2 All names that appear in data excerpts are pseudonyms.

3 Occasionally people who were not in the program were held to inhabit the
ecological space "out there" voluntarily. These people were usually cast as
predators or, at the very least, powerful enough to cope effectively with the
putatively savage vicissitudes of life on the streets. In this regard, see Sutter
(1966) for one of the classic discussions of the "righteous dope fiend" persona.
However, given the fact that their discussions took place in drug abuse treatment programs, my research subjects were heavily inclined to disapprove of
talk that "glorified" the drug life or that indicated faith in the possibility of
one's coping effectively with life "out there." Hence, people rarely spoke of
their *choosing* to "go out." Instead, returns to life "out there" were generally described as involuntary, that is, *addiction* induced.

4 I do not mean to suggest here that these four themes exhaustively describe
the opposition participants in my research settings discursively constructed
between the ecology of recovery and the ecology of addiction. Nor do I claim
that this ecological opposition was at all times uniformly endorsed by all program participants. My claim is only that these themes recurrently figured
prominently in members' discourse across all three settings and that they
demonstrate both that, and how, this ecological opposition was constructed.
Additionally, because the literature is already fairly replete with descriptions
of endogenous accounts of the ecology of recovery in drug abuse treatment
discourse (Bloor, McKeganey, and Fonkert 1988; Denzin 1993; Gubrium 1992;
Pollner and Stein 1996; Rubington 1977; Rudy 1986; Skoll 1992; Sugarman 1974;
Weinberg 1996; Weppner 1983; Wiseman 1970), my discussion is weighted decidedly in favor of describing how the ecology of addiction was itself depicted.

5 Two points merit notice here. First, though this image of the addict was, of
course, constructed in more and less (usually more) extreme guises, addiction
was *invariably* constructed as specifically antithetical to, rather than characteristic of, a given cultural order. Second, though this image is fiercely contested (and empirically tenuous), it is by no means exclusive to drug abuse
treatment discourse (Lindesmith 1940a). It may be found in journalistic ac-

counts, accounts proffered by drug warriors, family members of putative addicts, and others. Indeed, in his acclaimed ethnography *Crackhouse*, Terry
Williams (1992, 24–25) quotes one of his subjects, "Joan" (herself a heavy crack
user), as she describes the genuine crack addict: "The crack addict is the person who's lost all sense of what's going on. They are like zombies. They are out
there standing in the pouring rain. If it's cold and snowing, they'll be walking
up and down out there. They have no feelings. . . . It comes to the point where
they will set up family, friends, anybody—the point where they don't care
anymore."

6   Recalling the point made in note 3, occasionally nonprogram members were
held to persistently use drugs and to inhabit the space "out there" voluntarily.
However, program members overwhelmingly abstained from identifying
themselves, their peers in treatment, or, for that matter, anyone with whom
they empathized as one of these types of people. This was true for the obvious
reason that to do otherwise would undermine the assumption that people genuinely needed help. If people had been "out there" voluntarily, why would they
now be *struggling* to escape "the life" and therefore need therapeutic assistance
to help them do so?

7   It is routinely held among members of AA (and most others involved in addiction treatment) that addicts are often extremely ambivalent about admitting
they suffer from a disease that prevents them from controlling their drug use
(see Alcoholics Anonymous 2001). Hence, a widely acknowledged goal in drug
abuse treatment discourse is to break down the putative "denial" that keeps
the addicted person themselves unconsciously complicit with their disease. In
the interest of accomplishing this goal, a good deal of drug abuse treatment
discourse is taken up with inducing and offering confession of the depths to
which one's disease has forced one to sink (Denzin 1993; Rudy 1986; Weppner
1983).

8   It is worth mentioning that these accounts of collective descent are at least
partially confirmed by empirical research (Bourgois 1997; Currie 1993; Jencks
1994; Wacquant 1994, 1998; Wilson 1987). Though they may differ in their em-
phases of particular causal factors (a precipitous decline in manufacturing
jobs, state abandonment, capital flight, etc.), studies of urban poverty agree
that the circumstances of the urban poor in the United States have been getting more miserable, and in some instances more Hobbesian (see Wacquant
1998, 12–13), since the early 1970s. No doubt, program participants found each
other's accounts of a collective fall a bit more plausible for their relative parity
with the descending material conditions of contemporary urban poverty.

9   See Douglas (1966) for the classic statement concerning the cross-culturally
pervasive totemic imagery of cleanliness and dirtiness.

10 One reviewer interpreted my analysis as a case study of George Lakoff and
Mark Johnson's (1980) general arguments on the place of metaphor in human
discourse and cognition. I am not opposed to being linked with this tradition
but I would insist on two points. Lakoff and Johnson (1980, 5) write, "The es-

sence of metaphor is understanding and experiencing one kind of thing in terms of another." This formulation seems to imply some a priori resolutions as to the nature of the "kind of thing" that is being described such that literal terms of description might be somehow distinguished from metaphorical ones. I would prefer to avoid that implication here. Secondly, whereas Lakoff and Johnson (1980) demonstrate the importance of inherited narrative imagery as sense-making devices, they are not as concerned as I am to link the invocation of narrative imagery to specific types of shared work. I would argue that making sense of our experiences is only rarely, if ever, undertaken as an end in itself and is generally undertaken as a means of facilitating myriad other empirically identifiable kinds of work. Hence, for example, in the following section I explicitly distinguish making sense of our experiences in the academic context of social scientific work and making sense of our experiences in the *therapeutic* context of a drug abuse treatment program.

CHAPTER 5. THREE PROBLEMS WITH THE ADDICTION AS AKRASIA THESIS THAT ETHNOGRAPHY CAN SOLVE

An earlier version of this chapter appeared in *Against Better Judgment*, edited by Nick E. Evans and Patrick McKearney (Oxford: Berghahn Books, 2023), 50–69.

1 This is not a position uniformly adhered to in the literature concerning the addiction as akrasia thesis. Some prefer to see addiction as preference instability rather than a failure of one's actions to conform to stable preferences. This debate, while interesting, is not relevant to the arguments I am making in this chapter.

2 The Big Book was compiled by one of the cofounders of Alcoholics Anonymous, Bill W., and published for the first time in 1939 by Alcoholics Anonymous World Services. Its purpose was to outline the recovery program of Alcoholics Anonymous. It inaugurated the "Twelve Step Movement," which has arguably had more influence on thought and practice concerning recovery from addiction than any other popular or scientific movement in history. The Big Book has, since 1939, passed through three additional editions, sold more than thirty million copies, and been translated into more than seventy languages. In 2011, *Time* magazine listed it as one of the "best and most influential" one hundred nonfiction books published in English since its own founding in 1923. In 2012, the Big Book was named by the Library of Congress as one of the eighty-eight "Books That Shaped America."

3 All names are pseudonyms.

An earlier version of this chapter appeared in *Evaluating the Brain Disease
Model of Addiction*, edited by Nick Heather, Matt Field, Antony Moss, and
Sally Satel (London: Routledge, 2022), 373–83.

1 In the words of Harvard philosopher Richard Moran (2002, 211): "It is sometimes said that certain drugs 'produce' pleasure, but this is true only in the
same sense that either string quartets or ripe cheeses 'produce' pleasure. In
both cases we can provide the cause without producing the effect, because
the person exposed to either the drug or the music doesn't like it, doesn't see
what there is to enjoy in it. What was the very form of hazy, druggy pleasure
for someone else is for this person merely some unpleasant dizziness and
disorientation."

2 The brain disease literature is prone to uncritically reiterate a fairly narrow a
priori definition of self-control as executive function, response inhibition, or
impulse control and the loss of self-control as a submission to one's impulses.
Moving beyond a priori definitions, though, there are no compelling theoretical or empirical reasons to generically, or universally, equate disinhibition
with a loss of self-control, if by self-control we mean something like the rational pursuit of happiness. People often quite freely and deliberately use alcohol
or drugs to reduce their inhibitions without feeling, or inviting the accusation, that they have in any way forsaken their free agency or self-control. Autonomy, will, or self-control is exercised both through emotionally repressive
self-regulation and emotionally expressive self-revelation. Therapeutic self-
exploration, self-discovery, self-actualization, and empowerment overwhelmingly attend to both dimensions of who we are and what we do. If we are to
more fully understand addiction, we must understand that, and empirically
examine how, addictions pose a threat not only to our self-regulation but also
to our freedom more generally conceived. The ecological understanding of
addiction I am defending in this chapter does so in large part by juxtaposing
addiction and the much more commonly observed performance-enhancing
drug use.

3 Pickard (2013, 1146) writes in this regard: "Clinicians are able to hold service
users with disorders of agency responsible, indeed blameworthy, for harm,
without blaming them, because blame comes in two forms: detached and affective. Detached blame consists in judgments of blameworthiness, and may
further involve correspondingly appropriate revisions of intentions, the impo-
sition of negative consequences, and accountability and answerability. . . . Affective blame consists in negative reactions and emotions, whether rational or
not, which the blamer feels entitled to have. . . . Responsibility without blame
is responsibility without affective blame: without a sense of entitlement to any
negative reactive attitudes and emotions one might experience."

4 Here I rely on Rom Harré's (1987, 42) distinction between the *person* (understood as the "human being as a social individual embodied and publicly iden-

tifiable") and the *self* (understood as "that inner unity to which all personal experience [and I would add, conduct] belongs as attributes of a subject"). See also chapter 2, note 6.

5 As is discussed in chapter 2, I don't think brute determinism is confined to physical constraint.

6 This is made explicit in the following interview exchange:

> Foucault: Is it obvious that in liberating one's desires one will know how to behave ethically in pleasurable relationships with others?
> [Interviewer]: You say that liberty must be practiced ethically?
> Foucault: Yes, for what is morality, if not the practice of liberty, the deliberate practice of liberty?
> [Interviewer]: That means that you consider liberty as a reality already ethical in itself?
> Foucault: Liberty is the ontological condition of ethics. But ethics is the deliberate form assumed by liberty. (Foucault 1987, 115)

CHAPTER 7. POSTHUMANISM, ADDICTION, AND THE LOSS OF SELF-CONTROL: REFLECTIONS ON THE MISSING CORE IN ADDICTION SCIENCE

An earlier version of this chapter appeared in *International Journal of Drug Policy* 24, no. 3 (2013): 173–81.

1 Though one hears banter of "workaholics" and the like, in truth mere dedication to a form of activity or consumption is an extremely dubious stand-in for a genuine loss of self-control. The questions of whether this dedication is to a form of relief or pleasure, and whether it is virtuous or vicious, are clearly distinct from the question of whether it is voluntary or involuntary.

2 As noted in chapter 1, note 3, by "gross physiological withdrawal symptoms" I mean symptoms like vomiting, cramping, delirium tremens, runny nose, itchy eyes, in contrast to more diffuse effects of withdrawal like anxiety or headaches. The latter are less clearly reducible to specific physiological effects.

3 This tendency is not confined to the NIDA brain disease model but can also be seen elsewhere, as in the disinhibition literature (see Kallmen and Gustafson 1998; MacAndrew and Edgerton 1969). But there are no compelling theoretical or empirical reasons to universally equate disinhibition with a loss of self-control either. Many people deliberately use drugs quite happily and harmoniously to achieve precisely this effect without feeling, or inviting the accusation, that they have in any way forsaken their self-control.

4 Bourdieu's concept of habitus provides an illuminating analogy but is limited because he considered the habitus a strictly sociogenic set of sensibilities. Latour's notion of bodily articulation leaves open the possibility of a more theoretically porous regard for the range of possible influences on our embodied sensibilities (Weinberg 2021).

5 It should be remembered that while most people play a major role in assessing whether they are addicted, they rarely possess a monopoly on the right to do so. It is a straightforward matter, though, to study the empirical grounds on which people base their conclusions that *either they or others* have lost control of their drug use.

6 One reviewer worried that this argument reintroduces the transcendent liberal subject, as evaluative agent, that both I and posthumanist theorists more generally have been so concerned with avoiding. If we acknowledge that our various bodily articulations are often experienced and evaluated differently under different practical conditions, this worry should be averted. Indeed, putative addicts often, if not invariably, do struggle with the decision as to whether and to what extent they self-identify with their drug-using practices under different practical conditions.

Acker, Caroline Jean. 2002. *Creating the American Junkie: Addiction Research in the Classic Era of Narcotic Control*. Baltimore: Johns Hopkins University Press.

Agar, Michael. 1973. *Ripping and Running: A Formal Ethnography of Urban Heroin Addicts*. New York: Seminar Press.

Ainslie, George. 1992. *Picoeconomics*. Cambridge: Cambridge University Press.

Akers, Ronald L. 1992. *Drugs, Alcohol, and Society: Social Structure, Process, and Policy*. Belmont, CA: Wadsworth.

Alasuutari, Pertti. 1992. *Desire and Craving: A Cultural Theory of Alcoholism*. Albany: State University of New York Press.

Alcoholics Anonymous. 2001. *Alcoholics Anonymous: The Story of How Many Thousands of Men and Women Have Recovered from Alcoholism*. New York: Alcoholics Anonymous World Services.

Alexander, Bruce K. 2008. *The Globalization of Addiction*. Oxford: Oxford University Press.

Appleby, Joyce. 1992. *Liberalism and Republicanism in the Historical Imagination*. Cambridge, MA: Harvard University Press.

Bannister, Robert C. 1987. *Sociology and Scientism: The American Quest for Objectivity, 1880–1940*. Chapel Hill: University of North Carolina Press.

Baumeister, Roy F. 2003. "Ego Depletion and Self-Regulation Failure: A Resource Model of Self-Control." *Alcoholism: Clinical and Experimental Research* 27 (2): 281–84.

Baumohl, Jim, and Robin Room. 1987. "Inebriety, Doctors, and the State: Alcoholism Treatment Institutions before 1940." In *Recent Developments in Alcoholism*, vol. 5, edited by Marc Galanter, 135–74. New York: Plenum.

Baxter, Richard. (1673) 1825. *A Christian Directory*. London: Richard Edwards.

Becker, Gary S., and Kevin M. Murphy. 1988. "A Theory of Rational Addiction." *Journal of Political Economy* 96 (4): 675–700.

Becker, Howard S. 1953. "Becoming a Marijuana User." *American Journal of Sociology* 59:235–42.

Becker, Howard S. 1967. "History, Culture and Subjective Experience: An Explanation of Social Bases of Drug-Induced Experiences." *Journal of Health and Social Behavior* 8 (3): 163–76.

Berridge, Kent C. 2000. "Measuring Hedonic Impact in Animals and Infants: Microstructure of Affective Taste Reactivity Patterns." *Neuroscience and Biobehavioral Reviews* 24 (2): 173–98.

Berridge, Kent C. 2022. "Is Addiction a Brain Disease? The Incentive Sensitization View." In *Evaluating the Brain Disease Model of Addiction*, edited by Nick Heather, Matt Field, Sally Satel, and Antony Moss, 74–86. New York: Routledge.

Berry, Christopher J. 1994. *The Idea of Luxury*. Cambridge: Cambridge University Press.

Biernacki, Patrick. 1986. *Pathways from Heroin Addiction: Recovery without Treatment*. Philadelphia: Temple University Press.

Bloor, Michael, Neal McKeganey, and Dick Fonkert. 1988. *One Foot in Eden: A Sociological Study of the Range of Therapeutic Community Practice*. London: Routledge.

Blumer, Herbert. 1931. "Science without Concepts." *American Journal of Sociology* 36 (4): 515–33.

Blumer, Herbert. 1937. "Social Psychology." In *Man and Society*, edited by E. P. Schmidt, 144–98. New York: Prentice Hall.

Blumer, Herbert. 1969. *Symbolic Interactionism: Perspective and Method*. Berkeley: University of California Press.

Bogen, David, and Michael Lynch. 1993. "Do We Need a General Theory of Social Problems?" In *Reconsidering Social Constructionism: Debates in Social Problems Theory*, edited by James A. Holstein and Gale Miller, 213–37. New York: Aldine.

Bolton, David. 2010. "Conceptualisation of Mental Disorder and Its Personal Meanings." *Journal of Mental Health* 19 (4): 328–36.

Bourdieu, Pierre. 1975. "The Specificity of the Scientific Field and the Social Conditions for the Progress of Reason." *Social Science Information* 14 (5): 19–47.

Bourdieu, Pierre. 1990. *The Logic of Practice*. Stanford: Stanford University Press.

Bourdieu, Pierre. 2004. *Science of Science and Reflexivity*. Cambridge, UK: Polity.

Bourdieu, Pierre, and Loïc J. D. Wacquant. 1992. *An Invitation to Reflexive Sociology*. Chicago: University of Chicago Press.

Bourgois, Philippe. 1997. "In Search of Horatio Alger: Culture and Ideology in the Crack Economy." In *Crack in America: Demon Drugs and Social Justice*, edited by Craig Reinarman and Harry G. Levine, 57–76. Berkeley: University of California Press.

Bourgois, Philippe, and Jeff Schonberg. 2009. *Righteous Dopefiend*. Berkeley: University of California Press.

Breslau, Daniel. 2000. "Sociology after Humanism: A Lesson from Contemporary Science Studies." *Sociological Theory* 18 (2): 289–307.

Brown, L. Guy. 1931. "The Sociological Implications of Drug Addictions." *Journal of Educational Sociology* 4 (6): 358–69.

Brubaker, Rogers. 1993. "Social Theory as Habitus." In *Bourdieu: Critical Perspectives*, edited by Craig Calhoun, Edward LiPuma, and Moishe Postone, 212–34. Chicago: University of Chicago Press.

Burchell, Graham, Colin Gordon, and Peter Miller, eds. 1991. *The Foucault Effect.* Chicago: University of Chicago Press.

Callon, Michel. 1986. "Some Elements of a Sociology of Translation." In *Power, Action and Belief,* edited by John Law, 196–233. London: Routledge.

Calhoun, Craig. 1995. *Critical Social Theory: Culture, History and the Challenge of Difference.* Cambridge, MA: Blackwell.

Calhoun, Craig. 1998. "Explanation in Historical Sociology: Narrative, General Theory, and Historically Specific Theory." *American Journal of Sociology* 104 (3): 846–71.

Camic, Charles. 1986. "The Matter of Habit." *American Journal of Sociology* 91 (5): 1039–87.

Campbell, Nancy D. 2007. *Discovering Addiction: The Science and Politics of Substance Abuse Research.* Ann Arbor: University of Michigan Press.

Campbell, Nancy D. 2010. "Toward a Critical Neuroscience of 'Addiction.'" *BioSocieties* 5 (1): 89–104.

Carr, E. Summerson. 2011. *Scripting Addiction: The Politics of Therapeutic Talk and American Sobriety.* Princeton, NJ: Princeton University Press.

Childress, Anna Rose, Ronald Ehrman, Damaris J. Rohsenow, Steven J. Robbins, and Charles P. O'Brien. 1992. "Classically Conditioned Factors in Drug Dependence." In *Substance Abuse: A Comprehensive Text,* edited by Joyce H. Lowinson, Pedro Ruiz, Robert B. Millman, and John G. Langrad, 56–69. Baltimore: Williams and Wilkins.

Chodorow, Nancy J. 1999. *The Power of Feelings.* New Haven, CT: Yale University Press.

Cloward, Richard A., and Lloyd E. Ohlin. 1960. *Delinquency and Opportunity: A Theory of Delinquent Gangs.* New York: Free Press.

Collins, Harry M., and Steven Yearley. 1992. "Journey into Space." In *Science as Practice and Culture,* edited by Andrew Pickering, 369–89. Chicago: University of Chicago Press.

Conrad, Peter, and Joseph W. Schneider. 1992. *Deviance and Medicalization: From Badness to Sickness.* Philadelphia: Temple University Press.

Coulter, Jeff. 1994. "Is Contextualizing Necessarily Interpretive?" *Journal of Pragmatics* 21 (6): 689–98.

Coulter, Jeff, and E. D. Parsons. 1990. "The Praxiology of Perception: Visual Orientations and Practical Action." *Inquiry* 33 (3): 251–72.

Courtwright, David T. 2001. *Dark Paradise: A History of Opiate Addiction in America.* Cambridge, MA: Harvard University Press.

Courtwright, David T. 2010. "The NIDA Brain Disease Paradigm: History, Resistance, Spinoffs." *BioSocieties* 5 (1): 137–47.

Courtwright, David T. 2019. *The Age of Addiction: How Bad Habits Became Big Business.* Cambridge, MA: Harvard University Press.

Currie, Elliot. 1993. *Reckoning: Drugs, the Cities, and the American Future.* New York: Hill and Wang.

Dai, Bingham. 1937. *Opium Addiction in Chicago.* Shanghai: Commercial Press.

Daston, Lorraine. 2008. "On Scientific Observation." *Isis* 99 (1): 97–110.

Davidson, Donald. 1982. "Paradoxes of Irrationality." In *Philosophical Essays on Freud*, edited by Richard Wollheim and James Hopkins, 289–305. Cambridge: Cambridge University Press.

Davidson, Donald. 2001. *Essays on Actions and Events.* Oxford: Oxford University Press.

Davies, John Booth. 1992. *The Myth of Addiction.* Amsterdam: Harwood.

D'Elia, Donald J. 1974. *Benjamin Rush: Philosopher of the American Revolution.* Philadelphia: American Philosophical Society.

Dennis, Fay. 2019. *Injecting Bodies in More-than-Human Worlds.* London: Routledge.

Denzin, Norman K. 1993. *The Alcoholic Society: Addiction and Recovery of the Self.* New Brunswick, NJ: Transaction.

Dilkes-Frayne, Ella, Suzanne Fraser, Kiran Pienaar, and Renata Kokanovic. 2017. "Iterating 'Addiction': Residential Relocation and the Spatio-Temporal Production of Alcohol and Other Drug Consumption Patterns." *International Journal of Drug Policy* 44 (June): 164–73.

Douglas, Mary. 1966. *Purity and Danger: An Analysis of the Concepts of Pollution and Taboo.* London: Routledge and Kegan Paul.

Douglas, Mary, ed. 1987. *Constructive Drinking.* Cambridge: Cambridge University Press.

Dreyfus, Hubert L. 1991. *Being-in-the-World: A Commentary on Heidegger's "Being and Time," Division I.* Cambridge, MA: MIT Press.

Duff, Cameron. 2004. "Drug Use as a 'Practice of the Self': Is There Any Place for an 'Ethics of Moderation' in Contemporary Drug Policy?" *International Journal of Drug Policy* 15 (December): 385–93.

Duff, Cameron. 2008. "The Pleasure in Context." *International Journal of Drug Policy* 19 (October): 384–92.

Duster, Troy. 1970. *The Legislation of Morality: Law, Drugs and Moral Judgment.* New York: Free Press.

Edwards, Griffith. 2005. *Matters of Substance.* New York: St. Martin's.

Ekstrom, Laura Wadell. 2005. "Alienation, Autonomy, and the Self." *Midwest Studies in Philosophy* 29 (1): 45–67.

Elster, Jon. 1999. "Emotion and Addiction: Neurobiology, Culture, and Choice." In *Addiction*, edited by Jon Elster, 239–76. New York: Russell Sage Foundation.

Elster, Jon, and Ole-Jorgen Skog, eds. 1999. *Getting Hooked: Rationality and Addiction.* Cambridge: Cambridge University Press.

Evans, Jonathan. 2009. "How Many Dual-Process Theories Do We Need? One,

Two, or Many?" In *In Two Minds: Dual Processes and Beyond*, edited by Jonathan Evans and Keith Frankish, 33–54. Oxford: Oxford University Press.

Evans, Jonathan, and Keith Frankish, eds. 2009. *In Two Minds: Dual Processes and Beyond*. Oxford: Oxford University Press.

Faris, Robert E. L., and H. Warren Dunham. 1939. *Mental Disorders in Urban Areas: An Ecological Study of Schizophrenia and Other Psychoses*. Chicago: University of Chicago Press.

Ferentzy, Peter. 2001. "From Sin to Disease: Differences and Similarities between Past and Current Conceptions of Chronic Drunkenness." *Contemporary Drug Problems* 28 (3): 363–90.

Ferentzy, Peter. 2002. "Foucault and Addiction." *Telos* 125:167–91.

Fielding, Henry. 1751. *An Enquiry into the Causes of the Late Increase in Robbers*. London: A. Miller.

Finestone, Harold. 1957. "Cats, Kicks, and Color." *Social Problems* 5 (1): 3–13.

Foddy, Bennett, and Julian Savulescu. 2007. "Addiction Is Not an Affliction: Addictive Desires Are Merely Pleasure-Oriented Desires." *American Journal of Bioethics* 7 (1): 29–32.

Foddy, Bennett, and Julian Savulescu. 2010. "A Liberal Account of Addiction." *Philosophy, Psychiatry, and Psychology* 17 (1): 1–22.

Foucault, Michel. 1983. "The Subject and Power." In *Michel Foucault*, by Hubert L. Dreyfus and Paul Rabinow, 208–26. Chicago: University of Chicago Press.

Foucault, Michel. 1987. "The Ethic of Care for the Self as a Practice of Freedom: An Interview with Michel Foucault on January 20, 1984." *Philosophy and Social Criticism* 12 (2–3): 112–31.

Frankfurt, Harry G. 1999. *Necessity, Volition, and Love*. Cambridge: Cambridge University Press.

Frankish, Keith. 2009. "Systems and Levels: Dual System Theories and the Personal-Subpersonal Distinction." In *In Two Minds: Dual Processes and Beyond*, edited by Jonathan Evans and Keith Frankish, 89–108. Oxford: Oxford University Press.

Fraser, Suzanne, and David Moore, eds. 2011. *The Drug Effect: Health, Crime and Society*. Melbourne: Cambridge University Press.

Fraser, Suzanne, David Moore, and Helen Keane. 2014. *Habits: Remaking Addiction*. London: Palgrave Macmillan.

Fulford, K. W. M. 1989. *Moral Theory and Medical Practice*. Cambridge: Cambridge University Press.

Garcia, Angela. 2010. *The Pastoral Clinic: Addiction and Dispossession along the Rio Grande*. Berkeley: University of California Press.

Garfinkel, Harold. 1967. *Studies in Ethnomethodology*. Englewood Cliffs, NJ: Prentice-Hall.

Garland, Eric L., and Matthew O. Howard. 2018. "Mindfulness-Based Treatment of Addiction: Current State of the Field and Envisioning the Next Wave of Research." *Addiction Science and Clinical Practice* 13 (1): article no. 14.

Garriott, William, and Eugene Raikhel. 2015. "Addiction in the Making." *Annual Review of Anthropology* 44:477–91.

Gawin, Frank. 1991. "Cocaine Addiction: Psychology and Neurology." *Science* 251:1580–86.

Geertz, Clifford. 1973. *The Interpretation of Cultures: Selected Essays.* New York: Basic Books.

Giddens, Anthony, and Christopher Pierson. 1998. *Conversations with Anthony Giddens.* Stanford, CA: Stanford University Press.

Goffman, Erving. 1961. *Asylums: Essays on the Social Situations of Mental Patients and Other Inmates.* New York: Anchor Books.

Goldstein, Rita Z., and Nora D. Volkow. 2011. "Dysfunction of the Prefrontal Cortex in Addiction: Neuroimaging Findings and Clinical Implications." *Nature Reviews Neuroscience* 12:652–69.

Gomart, Emilie. 2002. "Towards a Generous Constraint: Freedom and Coercion in French Addiction Treatment." *Sociology of Health and Illness* 24 (5): 517–49.

Gomart, Emilie. 2004. "Surprised by Methadone: In Praise of Drug Substitution Treatment in a French Clinic." *Body and Society* 10 (2–3): 85–110.

Gomart, Emilie, and Antoine Hennion. 1999. "A Sociology of Attachment: Music Amateurs, Drug Users." In *Actor Network Theory and After*, edited by John Law and John Hassard, 220–47. Oxford: Blackwell.

Gowan, Teresa, and Sarah Whetstone. 2012. "Making the Criminal Addict: Subjectivity and Social Control in a Strong-Arm Rehab." *Punishment and Society* 14 (1): 69–93.

Granfeld, Robert, and Craig Reinarman, eds. 2015. *Expanding Addiction: Critical Essays.* London: Routledge.

Gubrium, Jaber F. 1992. *Out of Control: Family Therapy and Domestic Disorder.* Newbury Park, CA: Sage.

Gubrium, Jaber F., and James A. Holstein. 2009. "The Everyday Work and Auspices of Authenticity." In *Authenticity in Culture, Self and Society*, edited by Phillip Vannini and J. Patrick Williams, 121–38. Burlington, VT: Ashgate.

Hammersley, Martyn. 1989. *The Dilemma of Qualitative Method: Herbert Blumer and the Chicago Tradition.* London: Routledge.

Haraway, Donna J. 1991. *Symians, Cyborgs and Women: The Reinvention of Nature.* New York: Routledge.

Harre, Rom. 1987. "The Social Construction of Selves." In *Self and Identity*, edited by Krysia Yardley and Terry Honess, 41–52. New York: John Wiley and Sons.

Hayles, N. Katherine. 1999. *How We Became Posthuman.* Chicago: University of Chicago Press.

Heath, Dwight. 2012. *Drinking Occasions: Comparative Perspectives on Alcohol and Culture.* London: Routledge.

Heather, Nick. 2017. "Addiction as a Form of Akrasia." In *Addiction and Choice: Rethinking the Relationship*, edited by Nick Heather and Gabriel Segal, 133–50. Oxford: Oxford University Press.

Heather, Nick. 2020. "The Concept of Akrasia as the Foundation for a Dual Systems Theory of Addiction." *Behavioural Brain Research* 390 (July 15): article no. 112666.

Heather, Nick, Matt Field, Sally Satel, and Antony Moss, eds. 2022. *Evaluating the Brain Disease Model of Addiction.* New York: Routledge.

Heather, Nick, and Gabriel Segal. 2013. "Understanding Addiction: Donald Davidson and the Problem of Akrasia." *Addiction Research and Theory* 21 (6): 445–52.

Heather, Nick, and Gabriel Segal. 2015. "Is Addiction a Myth? Donald Davidson's Solution to the Problem of Akrasia Says Not." *International Journal of Alcohol and Drug Research* 4 (1): 77–83.

Heather, Nick, and Gabriel Segal, eds. 2017. *Addiction and Choice: Rethinking the Relationship.* Oxford: Oxford University Press.

Hellman, Matilda, Michael Egerer, Janne Stoneham, Sarah Forberger, Vilga Mannistolnkinen, Doris Ochterbeck, and Samantha Rundle. 2022. *Addiction and the Brain: Knowledge, Beliefs and Ethical Considerations from a Social Perspective.* Singapore: Palgrave Macmillan.

Henden, Edmund. 2017. "Addiction, Compulsion, and Weakness of the Will: A Dual-Process Perspective." In *Addiction and Choice: Rethinking the Relationship*, edited by Nick Heather and Gabriel Segal, 116–32. Oxford: Oxford University Press.

Heritage, John. 1984. *Garfinkel and Ethnomethodology.* Cambridge, UK: Polity.

Heyman, Gene. M. 2009. *Addiction: A Disorder of Choice.* Cambridge, MA: Harvard University Press.

Hochschild, Arlie R. 2012. *The Managed Heart.* 3rd ed. Berkeley: University of California Press.

Holstein, James A., and Jaber F. Gubrium. 1995. *The Active Interview.* Thousand Oaks, CA: Sage.

Holstein, James A., and Gale Miller. 1993. "Social Constructionism and Social Problems Work." In *Reconsidering Social Constructionism*, edited by James A. Holstein and Gale Miller, 151–72. Hawthorne, NY: Aldine de Gruyter.

Holton, Richard, and Kent Berridge. 2013. "Addiction between Compulsion and Choice." In *Addiction and Self-Control*, edited by Neil Levy, 239–68. Oxford: Oxford University Press.

Hughes, Kahryn. 2007. "Migrating Identities: The Relational Constitution of Drug Use and Addiction." *Sociology of Health and Illness* 29 (5): 673–91.

Hutchins, Edwin. 1995. *Cognition in the Wild.* Cambridge, MA: MIT Press.

Hyman, Steven E., Robert C. Malenka, and Eric J. Nestler. 2006. "Neural Mechanisms of Addiction: The Role of Reward-Related Learning and Memory." *Annual Review of Neuroscience* 29:565–98.

Jasanoff, Sheila. 2011. "The Practices of Objectivity in Regulatory Science." In *Social Knowledge in the Making*, edited by Charles Camic, Neil Gross, and Michele Lamont, 307–38. Chicago: University of Chicago Press.

Jencks, Christopher. 1994. *The Homeless.* Cambridge, MA: Harvard University Press.

Johnson, Bruce D. 1980. "Toward a Theory of Drug Subcultures." In *Theories on Drug Abuse: Selected Contemporary Perspectives*, edited by Dan J. Lettieri, Mollie Sayers, and Helen W. Pearson, 110–19. NIDA Research Monograph 30. Rockville, MD: National Institute on Drug Abuse.

Kalivas, Peter W., and Charles C. O'Brien. 2008. "Drug Addiction as a Pathology of Staged Neuroplasticity." *Neuropsychopharmacology* 33:166–80.

Kalivas, Peter W., and Nora D. Volkow. 2005. "The Neural Basis of Addiction: A Pathology of Motivation and Choice." *American Journal of Psychiatry* 162 (8): 1403–13.

Kallmen, Hakan, and Roland Gustafson. 1998. "Alcohol and Disinhibition." *European Addiction Research* 4:15–62.

Kandil, Hazem. 2022. "Power in Narrative and Narratives of Power in Historical Sociology." In *History in the Humanities and Social Sciences*, edited by Richard Bourke and Quentin Skinner, 141–64. Cambridge: Cambridge University Press.

Keane, Helen. 2002. *What's Wrong with Addiction?* New York: New York University Press.

Kelley, Ann E., and Kent C. Berridge. 2002. "The Neuroscience of Natural Rewards: Relevance to Addictive Drugs." *Journal of Neuroscience* 22 (9): 3306–11.

Knorr-Cetina, Karin. 1997. "Sociality with Objects: Social Relations in Postsocial Knowledge." *Theory, Culture and Society* 14 (4): 1–30.

Knott, Sarah. 2009. *Sensibility and the American Revolution*. Chapel Hill: University of North Carolina Press.

Koob, George F. 2006. "The Neurobiology of Addiction: A Neuroadaptational View Relevant for Diagnosis." *Addiction* 101 (September): 23–30.

Koob, George F., Luis Stinus, Michel Le Moal, and Floyd E. Bloom. 1989. "Opponent Process Theory of Motivation: Neurobiological Evidence from Studies of Opiate Dependence." *Neuroscience and Biobehavioral Reviews* 13 (2–3): 135–40.

Laidlaw, James. 2014. *The Subject of Virtue: An Anthropology of Ethics and Freedom*. Cambridge: Cambridge University Press.

Lakoff, George, and Mark Johnson. 1980. *Metaphors We Live By*. Chicago: University of Chicago Press.

Latour, Bruno. 1993. *We Have Never Been Modern*. Cambridge, MA: Harvard University Press.

Latour, Bruno. 1996. "On Interobjectivity." *Mind, Culture and Activity* 3 (4): 228–45.

Latour, Bruno. 2004. "How to Talk about the Body? The Normative Dimensions of Science Studies." *Body and Society* 10 (2–3): 205–29.

Latour, Bruno. 2005. *Reassembling the Social: An Introduction to Actor-Network Theory*. Oxford: Oxford University Press.

Law, John, and Vicky Singleton. 2005. "Object Lessons." *Organization* 12 (3): 331–55.

Leder, Drew. 1990. *The Absent Body*. Chicago: University of Chicago Press.

Leshner, Alan I. 1997. "Addiction Is a Brain Disease and It Matters." *Science* 278:45–47.

Levine, Donald N. 1995. *Visions of the Sociological Tradition*. Chicago: University of Chicago Press.

Levine, Harry G. 1978. "The Discovery of Addiction: Changing Conceptions of Habitual Drunkenness in America." *Journal of Studies on Alcohol* 39 (1): 143–74.

Levy, Neil. 2005. "Autonomy and Addiction." *Canadian Journal of Philosophy* 36 (3): 427–48.

Levy, Neil, ed. 2013. *Addiction and Self Control: Perspectives from Philosophy, Psychology and Neuroscience*. Oxford: Oxford University Press.

Lewis, J. David, and Richard L. Smith. 1980. *American Sociology and Pragmatism: Mead, Chicago Sociology, and Symbolic Interaction*. Chicago: University of Chicago Press.

Lewis, Marc. 2015. *The Biology of Desire: Why Addiction Is Not a Disease*. New York: Public Affairs.

Lewis, Marc. 2017a. "Addiction and the Brain: Development, Not Disease." *Neuroethics* 10 (1): 7–18.

Lewis Marc. 2017b. "Choice Isn't Simple. Reply to Pickard." *Neuroethics* 10 (1): 181–83.

Lewis Marc. 2017c. "A Graded Approach to 'Disease'—Help or Hindrance? Reply to Berridge." *Neuroethics* 10 (1): 35–37.

Lewis, Marc. 2018. "Brain Change in Addiction as Learning, Not Disease." *New England Journal of Medicine* 379 (16): 1551–60.

Lindesmith, Alfred R. 1938a. "Rejoinder" [to Slight 1938]. *American Journal of Sociology* 43 (4): 611–13.

Lindesmith, Alfred R. 1938b. "A Sociological Theory of Drug Addiction" [including Slight 1938 and Lindesmith 1938b]. *American Journal of Sociology* 43 (4): 593–613.

Lindesmith, Alfred R. 1940a. "Dopefiend Mythology." *Journal of Criminal Law, Criminology and Police Science* 31 (July–August): 199–208.

Lindesmith, Alfred R. 1940b. "The Drug Addict as Psychopath." *American Sociological Review* 5:914–20.

Lindesmith, Alfred R. 1947. *Opiate Addiction*. Bloomington, IN: Principia Press.

Lindesmith, Alfred R. 1960. "Social Problems and Sociological Theory." *Social Problems* 8 (2): 98–102.

Lindesmith, Alfred R. 1965a. *The Addict and the Law*. Bloomington: Indiana University Press.

Lindesmith, Alfred R. 1965b. "Problems in the Social Psychology of Addiction." In *Narcotics*, edited by Daniel M. Wilner and Gene G. Kassenbaum, 118–39. New York: McGraw-Hill.

Lindesmith, Alfred R. 1968. *Addiction and Opiates*. Chicago: Aldine.

Lindesmith, Alfred R., and Anselm L. Strauss. *Social Psychology*. Rev. ed. New York: Holt, Rinehart and Winston, 1956.

Longino, Helen E. 2002. *The Fate of Knowledge*. Princeton, NJ: Princeton University Press.

Loseke, Donileen R. 1999. *Thinking about Social Problems: An Introduction to Constructionist Perspectives*. New York: Aldine de Gruyter.

MacAndrew, Craig, and Robert Edgerton. 1969. *Drunken Comportment*. Chicago: Aldine.

Marlatt, G. Alan, and Judith R. Gordon, eds. 1985. *Relapse Prevention: Maintenance Strategies in the Treatment of Addictive Behaviors*. New York: Guilford Press.

Marvasti, Amir. 1998. "'Homelessness' as Narrative Redemption." *Perspectives on Social Problems* 10:167–82.

Marx, Karl. 1978. *Economic and Philosophical Manuscripts*. In *The Marx-Engels Reader*, edited by Robert C. Tucker, 66–125. 2nd ed. New York: W. W. Norton.

Matza, David. 1969. *Becoming Deviant*. Englewood Cliffs, NJ: Prentice-Hall.

Maynard, Douglas W., and John Heritage, eds. 2022. *The Ethnomethodological Program: Legacies and Prospects*. Oxford: Oxford University Press.

McAuliffe, William E., and Robert A. Gordon. 1974. "A Test of Lindesmith's Theory of Addiction: The Frequency of Euphoria among Long-Term Addicts." *American Journal of Sociology* 79 (4): 795–840.

Merleau-Ponty, Maurice. 1962.*The Phenomenology of Perception*. London: Routledge and Kegan Paul.

Merton, Robert. 1938. "Social Structure and Anomie." *American Sociological Review* 3 (5): 672–82.

Metzl, Jonathan M., and Anna Kirkland, eds. 2010. *Against Health: How Health Became the New Morality*. New York: New York University Press.

Mill, John Stuart. (1859) 2005. *On Liberty*. New York: Cosimo.

Mills, C. Wright. 1940. "Situated Actions and Vocabularies of Motive." *American Sociological Review* 5 (6): 904–13.

Mills, C. Wright. 1943. "The Professional Ideology of the Social Pathologists." *American Journal of Sociology* 49 (2): 165–80.

Mol, Annemarie. 2002. *The Body Multiple: Ontology in Medical Practice*. Durham, NC: Duke University Press.

Mol, Annemarie, and John Law. 2004. "Embodied Action, Enacted Bodies: The Example of Hypoglycaemia." *Body and Society* 10 (2–3): 43–62.

Moore, David. 2004. "Beyond 'Subculture' in the Ethnography of Illicit Drug Use." *Contemporary Drug Problems* 31 (2): 181–212.

Moran, Richard. 2002. "Frankfurt on Identification: Ambiguities of Activity in Mental Life." In *Contours of Agency: Essays on Themes from Harry Frankfurt*, edited by Sarah Buss and Lee Overton, 189–217. Cambridge, MA: MIT Press.

Müller, Christian P., and Gunter Schumann. 2011. "Drugs as Instruments: A New Framework for Non-addictive Psychoactive Drug Use." *Behavioral and Brain Sciences* 34 (6): 293–310.

Musto, David F. 1987. *The American Disease: Origins of Narcotic Control*. Expanded ed. New York: Oxford University Press.

Netherland, Julie, ed. 2012. *Critical Perspectives on Addiction*. Bingley, UK: Emerald.

Nettleton, Sarah, Jo Neale, and Lucy Pickering. 2011. "'I Don't Think There's Much of a Rational Mind in a Drug Addict when They Are in the Thick of It': Towards an Embodied Analysis of Recovering Heroin Users." *Sociology of Health and Illness* 33 (3): 341–55.

Nichols, John R. 1965. "How Opiates Change Behavior." *Scientific American* 212 (2): 80–88.

Nicholls, James. 2009. *The Politics of Alcohol: A History of the Drink Question in England*. Manchester: Manchester University Press.

Nussbaum, Martha. 2006. *Frontiers of Justice: Disability, Nationality, Species Membership*. Cambridge, MA: Harvard University Press.

O'Brien, Charles P., Nora Volkow, and T. K. Li. 2006. "What's in a Word? Addiction versus Dependence in DSM V." *American Journal of Psychiatry* 163 (5): 764–65.

O'Malley, Pat, and Mariana Valverde. 2004. "Pleasure, Freedom and Drugs: The Uses of 'Pleasure' in Liberal Governance of Drug and Alcohol Consumption." *Sociology* 38 (1): 25–42.

Orphanides, Athanasios, and David Zervos. 1995. "Rational Addiction with Learning and Regret." *Journal of Political Economy* 103 (4): 739–58.

Ostrow, James M. 1990. *Social Sensitivity: A Study of Habit and Experience*. Albany: State University of New York Press.

Peele, Stanton. 1989. *Diseasing of America*. Lexington, MA: Lexington Books.

Pickard, Hanna. 2013. "Responsibility without Blame: Philosophical Reflections on Clinical Practice." In *Oxford Handbook of Philosophy and Psychiatry*, edited by K. W. M. Fulford, Martin Davies, Richard G. T. Gipps, George Graham, John Sadler, Giovanni Stanghellini, and Tim Thornton, 1134–52. Oxford: Oxford University Press.

Pickard, Hanna. 2017. "Responsibility without Blame for Addiction." *Neuroethics* 10 (1): 169–80.

Pickering, Andrew. 1993. "The Mangle of Practice: Agency and Emergence in the Sociology of Science." *American Journal of Sociology* 99 (3): 559–89.

Pickering, Andrew. 1995. *The Mangle of Practice*. Chicago: University of Chicago Press.

Pittman, David J., and Calvin Wayne Gordon. 1958. *Revolving Door: A Study of the Chronic Police Case Inebriate*. New Haven, CT: Yale University Press.

Pocock, J. G. A. 1975. *The Machiavellian Moment: Florentine Political Thought and the Atlantic Republican Tradition*. Princeton, NJ: Princeton University Press.

Polanyi, Michael. 1962. *Personal Knowledge: Towards a Post-critical Philosophy*. Chicago: University of Chicago Press.

Pollner, Melvin, and Jill Stein. 1996. "Narrative Mapping of Social Worlds: The Voice of Experience in Alcoholics Anonymous." *Symbolic Interaction* 19 (3): 203–23.

Porter, Roy. 1985. "The Drinking Man's Disease: The 'Pre-history' of Alcoholism in Georgian Britain." *British Journal of Addiction* 80 (4): 385–96.

Porter, Roy. 1992. "Addicted to Modernity: Nervousness in the Early Consumer Society." In *Culture in History*, edited by Joseph Melling and Jonathan Barry, 180–94. Exeter: Exeter University Press.

Preble, Edward, and John J. Casey. 1969. "Taking Care of Business: The Heroin User's Life on the Street." *International Journal of the Addictions* 4 (1): 1–24.

Raikhel, Eugene. 2016. *Governing Habits: Treating Alcoholism in the Post-Soviet Clinic*. Ithaca, NY: Cornell University Press.

Raikhel, Eugene, and William Garriott, eds. 2013. *Addiction Trajectories*. Durham, NC: Duke University Press.

Ray, Marsh. 1961. "The Cycle of Abstinence and Relapse among Heroin Addicts." *Social Problems* 9 (2): 132–40.

Reinarman, Craig. 2005. "Addiction as Accomplishment: The Discursive Construction of Disease." *Addiction Research and Theory* 13 (4): 307–20.

Reinarman, Craig. 2013. "On the Cultural Domestication of Intoxicants." In *Intoxication and Society: Problematic Pleasures of Drugs and Alcohol,* edited by Jon Herring, Ciaran Regan, Darin Weinberg, and Phil Withington, 153–71. London: Palgrave Macmillan.

Reinarman, Craig, and Harry G. Levine, eds. 1997. *Crack in America: Demon Drugs and Social Justice*. Berkeley: University of California Press, 1997.

Reith, Gerda. 2004. "Consumption and Its Discontents: Addiction, Identity and the Problems of Freedom." *British Journal of Sociology* 55 (2): 283–300.

Reith, Gerda. 2019. *Addictive Consumption: Capitalism, Modernity and Excess*. London: Routledge.

Robins, Lee N. 1993. "Vietnam Veterans' Rapid Recovery from Heroin Addiction: A Fluke or Normal Expectation?" *Addiction* 88:1041–54.

Robinson, Terry E., and Kent C. Berridge. 2003. "Addiction." *Annual Review of Psychology* 54 (February): 25–53.

Rojeberg, Ole. 2004. "Taking Absurd Theories Seriously: Economics and the Case of Rational Addiction Theories." *Philosophy of Science* 71 (3): 263–85.

Room, Robin. 1976. "Ambivalence as a Sociological Explanation: The Case of Cultural Explanations of Alcohol Problems." *American Sociological Review* 41 (6): 1047–65.

Room, Robin. 1983. "Sociological Aspects of the Disease Concept of Alcoholism." *Research Advances in Alcohol and Drug Problems* 7:47–91.

Room, Robin. 1984. "Alcohol and Ethnography: A Case of Problem Deflation?" *Current Anthropology* 25 (2): 169–78.

Room, Robin. 1985. "Dependence and Society." *British Journal of Addiction* 80 (2): 133–39.

Rorty, Richard. 1979. *Philosophy and the Mirror of Nature*. Princeton, NJ: Princeton University Press.

Rorty, Richard. 1991. *Objectivity, Relativism and Truth*. Cambridge: Cambridge University Press.

Rose, Nikolas. 1990. *Governing the Soul*. London: Routledge.

Rose, Nikolas, Pat O'Malley, and Mariana Valverde. 2006. "Governmentality." *Annual Review of Law and Social Science* 2 (December): 83–104.

Rosenbaum, Marsha. 1981. *Women on Heroin*. New Brunswick, NJ: Rutgers University Press.

Rosenberg, Charles E. 1992. *Explaining Epidemics: And Other Studies in the History of Medicine.* Cambridge: Cambridge University Press.

Rouse, Joseph. 2002. *How Scientific Practices Matter.* Chicago: University of Chicago Press.

Rouse, Timothy P., and N. Prabha Unnithan. 1993. "Comparative Ideologies and Alcoholism: The Protestant and Proletarian Ethics." *Social Problems* 40 (2): 213–27.

Rubington, Earl. 1968. "The Bottle Gang." *Quarterly Journal of Studies on Alcohol* 29 (4): 943–55.

Rubington, Earl. 1977. "The Role of the Halfway House in the Rehabilitation of Alcoholics." In *The Biology of Alcoholism*, vol. 5, *Treatment and Rehabilitation of the Chronic Alcoholic*, edited by Benjamin Kissin and Henri Beglieter, 351–83. New York: Plenum.

Rudy, David R. 1986. *Becoming Alcoholic: Alcoholics Anonymous and the Reality of Alcoholism.* Carbondale: Southern Illinois University Press.

Runes, Dagobert D., ed. 1947. *The Selected Writings of Benjamin Rush.* New York: Philosophical Library.

Ryan, Richard M., and Edward L. Deci. 2001. "On Happiness and Human Potentials: A Review of Research on Hedonic and Eudaimonic Well-Being." *Annual Review of Psychology* 52 (February): 141–66.

SAMHSA (Substance Abuse and Mental Health Services Administration), Office of Applied Studies. 2008. *The NSDUH Report: Substance Use and Dependence Following Initiation of Alcohol or Illicit Drug Use.* Rockville, MD: Department of Health and Human Services.

Satel, Sally, and Scott O. Lilienfeld. 2013. *Brainwashed: The Seductive Appeal of Mindless Neuroscience.* New York: Basic Books.

Saunders, Clare, and David E. Over. 2009. "In Two Minds about Rationality?" In *In Two Minds: Dual Processes and Beyond*, edited by Jonathan Evans and Keith Frankish, 317–34. Oxford: Oxford University Press.

Schmidt, Laura A. 1995. "'A Battle Not Man's but God's': Origins of the American Temperance Crusade in the Struggle for Religious Authority." *Journal of Studies on Alcohol* 56 (1): 110–21.

Schneider, Joseph W. 1978. "Deviant Drinking as Disease: Alcoholism as Social Accomplishment." *Social Problems* 25 (4): 361–72.

Schull, Natasha D. 2012. *Addiction by Design: Machine Gambling in Las Vegas.* Princeton, NJ: Princeton University Press.

Sedgwick, Eve Kosofsky. 1993. "Epidemics of the Will." In *Tendencies*, 130–41. Durham, NC: Duke University Press.

Shusterman, Richard. 1991. "Beneath Interpretation." In *The Interpretive Turn: Philosophy, Science, Culture*, edited by David R. Hiley, James F. Bohman, and Richard Shusterman, 102–28. Ithaca, NY: Cornell University Press.

Singer, Merrill C. 2012. "Anthropology and Addiction: An Historical Review." *Addiction* 107 (10): 1747–55.

Skoll, Geoffrey R. 1992. *Walk the Walk and Talk the Talk: An Ethnography of a Drug Abuse Treatment Facility.* Philadelphia: Temple University Press.

Slight, David. 1938. "Comment" [on Lindesmith 1938b]. *American Journal of Sociology* 43 (4): 610–11.

Starr, Paul. 1982. *The Social Transformation of American Medicine: The Rise of a Sovereign Profession and the Making of a Vast Industry*. New York: Basic Books.

Stephens, Richard C. 1991. *The Street Addict Role: A Theory of Heroin Addiction*. Albany: State University of New York Press.

Straus, Robert. 1946. "Alcohol and the Homeless Man." *Quarterly Journal of Studies on Alcohol* 7 (3): 360–404.

Sugarman, Barry. 1974. *Daytop Village: A Therapeutic Community*. New York: Holt, Rinehart and Winston.

Sutter, Alan G. 1966. "The World of the Righteous Dope Fiend." *Issues in Criminology* 2 (2): 177–223.

Sutter, Alan G. 1969. "Worlds of Drug Use on the Street Scene." In *Delinquency, Crime, and Social Process*, edited by D. R. Cressey and D. A. Ward, 802–29. New York: Harper and Row.

Swedberg, Richard. 2018. "How to Use Max Weber's Ideal Type in Sociological Analysis." *Journal of Classical Sociology* 18 (3): 181–96.

Szasz, Thomas. 2003. *Ceremonial Chemistry*. Rev. ed. Syracuse, NY: Syracuse University Press.

Taylor, Charles. 1989. *Sources of the Self: The Making of the Modern Identity*. Cambridge, MA: Harvard University Press.

Taylor, Charles. 1993. "To Follow a Rule." In *Bourdieu: Critical Perspectives*, edited by Craig Calhoun, Edward LiPuma, and Moishe Postone, 45–60. Chicago: University of Chicago Press.

Thomas, Keith. 1971. *Religion and the Decline of Magic*. Oxford: Oxford University Press.

Turner, Bryan S. 2018. "(I Can't Get No) Satisfaction: Happiness and Successful Societies." *Journal of Sociology* 54 (3): 279–93.

Turner, Ralph H. 1976. "The Real Self: From Institution to Impulse." *American Journal of Sociology* 81 (5): 989–1016.

Turner, Stephen. 1994. *The Social Theory of Practices: Tradition, Tacit Knowledge and Presuppositions*. Chicago: University of Chicago Press.

Valverde, Mariana. 1998. *Diseases of the Will: Alcohol and the Dilemmas of Freedom*. Cambridge: Cambridge University Press.

Volkow, Nora D., George F. Koob, and A. Thomas McLellan. 2016. "Neurobiologic Advances from the Brain Disease Model of Addiction." *New England Journal of Medicine* 37 (4): 363–71.

Vrecko, Scott. 2010. "Birth of a Brain Disease: Science, the State, and Addiction Neuropolitics." *History of the Human Sciences* 23 (4): 52–67.

Wacquant, Loïc. 1994. "The New Urban Color Line: The State and Fate of the Ghetto in Post Fordist America." In *Social Theory and the Politics of Identity*, edited by Craig Calhoun, 231–76. Oxford: Blackwell.

Wacquant, Loïc. 1998. "Inside the Zone: The Social Art of the Hustler in the Black American Ghetto." *Theory, Culture, and Society* 15 (2): 1–36.

Wacquant, Loïc. 2016. "A Concise Genealogy and Anatomy of Habitus." *Sociological Review* 64 (1): 64–72.

Waldorf, Dan. 1983. "Natural Recovery from Opiate Addiction: Some Social Psychological Processes of Untreated Recovery." *Journal of Drug Issues* 13 (2): 237–80.

Waldorf, Dan, Craig Reinarman, and Sheigla Murphy. 1991. *Cocaine Changes: The Experience of Using and Quitting.* Philadelphia: Temple University Press.

Warner, Jessica. 1994. "'Resolv'd to Drink No More': Addiction as a Preindustrial Construct." *Journal of Studies on Alcohol* 55 (6): 685–91.

Waterston, Alisse. 1993. *Street Addicts in the Political Economy.* Philadelphia: Temple University Press.

Weinberg, Darin. 1996. "The Enactment and Appraisal of Authenticity in a Skid Row Therapeutic Community." *Symbolic Interaction* 19 (2): 137–62.

Weinberg, Darin. 1997. "Lindesmith on Addiction: A Critical History of a Classic Theory." *Sociological Theory* 15 (2): 150–61.

Weinberg, Darin. 2000a. "'Out There': The Ecology of Addiction in Drug Abuse Treatment Discourse." *Social Problems* 47 (4): 606–21.

Weinberg, Darin. 2000b. "Self-Empowerment in Two Therapeutic Communities." In *Institutional Selves: Troubled Identities in a Postmodern World,* edited by Jaber F. Gubrium and James A. Holstein, 84–104. Oxford: Oxford University Press.

Weinberg, Darin. 2005. *Of Others Inside: Insanity, Addiction, and Belonging in America.* Philadelphia: Temple University Press.

Weinberg, Darin. 2014. *Contemporary Social Constructionism: Key Themes.* Philadelphia: Temple University Press.

Weinberg, Darin. 2021. "Diagnosis as Topic and as Resource: Reflections on the Epistemology and Ontology of Disease in Medical Sociology." *Symbolic Interaction* 44 (2): 367–91.

Weppner, Robert S. 1983. *The Untherapeutic Community: Organizational Behavior in a Failed Addiction Treatment Program.* Lincoln: University of Nebraska Press.

West, Robert. 2006. *Theory of Addiction.* Oxford: Blackwell.

Wiener, Carolyn L. 1981. *The Politics of Alcoholism: Building an Arena around a Social Problem.* New Brunswick, NJ: Transaction Books.

Williams, Terry. 1992. *Crackhouse: Notes from the End of the Line.* Reading, MA: Addison-Wesley.

Wilson, William Julius. 1987. *The Truly Disadvantaged: The Inner City, the Underclass, and Public Policy.* Chicago: University of Chicago Press.

Winick, Charles. 1962. "Maturing Out of Narcotic Addiction." *Bulletin on Narcotics* 14 (5): 1–7.

Wiseman, Jacqueline P. 1970. *Stations of the Lost: The Treatment of Skid Row Alcoholics.* Englewood Cliffs, NJ: Prentice Hall.

Withington, Phil. 2007. "Public Discourse, Corporate Citizenship, and State Formation in Early Modern England." *American Historical Review* 112 (4): 1016–38.

Wittgenstein, Ludwig. 1953. *Philosophical Investigations*. Oxford: Basil Blackwell.

Wittgenstein, Ludwig. 1958. *The Blue and Brown Books*. Oxford: Blackwell.

Wood, Gordon S. 1998. *The Creation of the American Republic, 1776–1787*. Chapel Hill: University of North Carolina Press.

Zigon, Jarrett. 2007. "Moral Breakdown and Ethical Demand: A Theoretical Framework for an Anthropology of Moralities." *Anthropological Theory* 7 (2): 131–50.

Zigon, Jarrett. 2011. *"HIV Is God's Blessing": Rehabilitating Morality in Neoliberal Russia*. Berkeley: University of California Press.

Zigon, Jarrett. 2019. *A War on People: Drug Use Politics and a New Ethics of Community*. Oakland: University of California Press.

Zinberg, Norman E. 1984. *Drug, Set, and Setting: The Basis for Controlled Intoxicant Use*. New Haven, CT: Yale University Press.

culture, ix, 17, 42–43, 56, 74, 101, 104–5, 107, 135, 139, 150, 153; addiction as culture bound phenomenon, 33–37; and ecology of addiction, 82, 159n1, 159n5; liberalism and popular culture, 59, 60, 117, 119; and nature, 9–11, 124, 134; of Protestants, 54–55; and recovery, 77–96, 113; and science, vii, 18–19, 140, 158n2; subcultures, 28, 30–31, 48, 92

Daston, Lorraine, 16
Davidson, Donald, 4, 97, 114; on akrasia, 99–100; on partitioning of the mind, 110–11; on principle of charity and mental holism, 111–12, 113
Davies, John B., 17, 35, 42, 48, 49, 107
degeneracy, 118, 131–32
Denzin, Norman K., 30, 31, 72, 78, 136, 158n3
desire, 7, 27, 46, 57, 58, 62, 105–6, 116, 123; on biology of, 119, 126; Foucault on, 163n6; Frankfurt on, 108; and hedonic values, 40, 60–61, 157n7; Lindesmith on, 67–68; as want, 45, 133
determinism, 3–4, 50, 163n5; biological/ neurological, 10, 21, 31, 36, 39, 44–47, 59, 61, 101, 134, 140–42; Foucault on, 123, 124–25; Goffman on, 43–44; psychological, 10, 31, 68–70, 151; social structural, 20, 29, 31, 64–65; in contrast to slavery, 40, 60, 157n5
Diagnostic and Statistical Manual of Mental Disorders (DSM), 14
disease, 16, 36–37, 49–50, 51–52, 53–54, 57; Mol on, 143–44; early modern Protestant understanding of, 54–55; and type/token problem, 93
disease theory of addiction, 51, 54, 75, 78, 84, 99, 130–32, 159n1; and Alcoholics Anonymous, 160n7; and the brain, 3, 17, 44–47, 61; and loss of self-control, 45–47, 51, 61–62, 77, 82, 162n2; and luxury, 58; and posthumanism, 36–37, 139–48; and rationality, 93–95; and sinful madness, 54, 55; as universal and value free, 43, 59, 134; and unnatural rewards, 44–45, 59; as warrant for sympathy, 40, 92–93, 115–16, 119–21

Douglas, Mary, 17, 107, 160n9
dual systems/processes theory, 101–14
Duff, Cameron, 42, 137, 145
Durkheim, Emile, 66, 116, 117
Duster, Troy, 34, 135

ecology of addiction, 21–22, 77–78, 80–96, 115–28, 159n1, 159n3, 159n4, 162n2; and brain disease theory of addiction, 119–21; and choice theory, 121–23; divided habitus and self-actualization, 125–28
Edwards, Griffith, 45
Elster, Jon, 33, 95
emotion, 71, 88, 104, 119, 131, 136, 162n3; rationality and, 7–9; and restraint as self-control, 22, 46, 98, 105–9, 114, 162n2
Enlightenment, 54–55; Scottish, 60
ethics, 2, 3, 44, 47, 50, 54, 60, 104, 105, 114, 130, 156n5, 156n1, 157n7; and accountability, 17–18, 20, 43–44, 62, 121; Foucault on, 4, 123–25, 128, 163n6; and science, 6–7
ethnography, viii, 2, 6, 10, 11, 17, 19, 20, 30, 34, 42, 77–96, 100–1, 103–14, 156n1
ethnomethodology, 2, 6–7, 15–16
eudaemonic values, 40, 61, 157n7
executive function, 46, 103, 105, 106, 139, 162n2
experience, 10, 17, 44, 49, 112, 137, 158n2, 160–61n10; of addiction and recovery, viii, 2, 34, 36, 60, 74–75, 100–101, 103, 132; of drug effects, 12, 26, 30, 72, 74, 106, 107, 119–20, 126, 138, 141, 145; Fleck on, 16; of freedom, 40, 61, 133, 134; Lindesmith on, 63–64, 67, 68, 70, 150, 152–53; of loss of self-control, 80–96, 125–28; of mental affliction, 59, 61–62; praxiological approach to the meaning of, 5, 29, 73, 75, 126, 153

Ferentzy, Peter, 33, 53
Fielding, Henry (18th-century writer), 57
Foddy, Bennett, 47, 48, 49
Foucault, Michel, 131; on freedom and ethics, 4, 123–25, 128, 163n6
Frankfurt, Harry G., 4, 5, 8, 107–9, 114
Fraser, Suzanne, 42, 47, 135
freedom, 3–4, 10, 18, 36, 39–62, 106, 107, 114, 117, 122, 128, 130, 145, 151, 153–54,

157n5, 162n2; Foucault on, 4, 123–25, 163n6; Frankfurt on, 4, 5, 8, 107–9
free will, 3–4, 52, 53, 55, 109, 125, 157n5. *See also* freedom
functionalism, 28–29, 30

Galliher, John F., 149–54
Garcia, Angela, 42
Garfinkel, Harold, vii, 6, 15, 16, 29
Garriot, William, 42, 46
Geertz, Clifford, 10, 159n1
generalizing science, viii, 3–4, 6–7, 11–12, 13, 39–62, 65, 97–114, 140–42, 147, 156n1, 162n2; Bourdieu and, 19
Giddens, Anthony, 50
Goffman Erving, 43–44
Gomart, Emilie, 34, 36, 142, 143
governmentality, 123–25
Gowan, Teresa, 42, 43
Gubrium, Jaber F., 35, 96, 159n4

habit, 5, 8, 13, 52, 54, 57, 62, 102, 104, 127, 128, 131, 141; Fleck and Garfinkel on 15–16; nonpathological, 15–16, 106, 126; in 20th-century American sociology, 66–67
habitus, 5, 74, 142, 153–54; divided, 125–28; as exclusively sociogenic, 163n4
Haraway, Donna J., 11, 35, 139–40
Harre, Rom, 157n6
Heath, Dwight B., 42
Heather, Nick, 3, 32, 39, 48, 49, 106, 121; on akrasia, 98–102
hedonic values, 40, 61, 120, 157n7
Hellman, Matilde, 34
Heyman, Gene M., 39, 48, 49, 118, 121
historicism, 18–19, 41
history, vii, viii, ix, 2, 6, 10, 20; of addiction science, 39–62, 116–19, 130–39; and American pragmatism, 13–14; of drug policy, 25; Foucault and freedom, 123–25; of Lindesmith's theory of addiction, 64–71; of science, 18–19, 140, 158n2; and social constructionism, 33–34; of social problems theory, 91; universals as immune to, 11, 12, 19
Holstein, James A., 35, 78, 83, 93, 96

homelessness, 86, 87, 89, 112, 113; and drug use, 79, 84, 85, 92, 93, 95–96, 112
Hughes, Kahryn, 48, 136–37, 138–39, 144
human nature, 35, 111, 117, 134, 139
Hutchins, Edwin, 40, 105
Hyman, Steven E., 44, 49, 157n2
"hyperbolic discounting" of the future, by addicts, 8, 32, 121, 127

incentives, viii, 83, 95, 115, 123. *See also* punishment; reward
incentive sensitivity, 3, 99, 121; rational choice, plants and, 48
incentive sensitization theory, 45–46, 127, 141

Kalivas, Peter W., 45, 46, 106
Keane, Helen, 33, 47, 135
Knorr-Cetina, Karin, 11, 35, 139
Koob, George F., 39, 45, 133

Laidlaw, James, 19, 104, 106, 156n1
Latour, Bruno, 5, 11, 26, 35, 139, 143; and bodily articulation, 36–37, 140, 141–42, 144–46, 163n4; and culture/nature dichotomy, 10; and learning to be affected by external stimuli, 36–37, 140–42; silence on multiplicity of the body, 142, 144; and subjective/objective dichotomy, 140–41
Leshner, Alan I., 40, 132
Levine, Harry Gene, 17, 33, 34, 51, 52, 77, 89, 92, 129, 130, 135
Levy, Neil, 102, 106, 121
Lewis, Marc, 39, 48, 49, 50, 120, 121, 126; on competing synaptic networks, 62; on neurological distortion of cognitive functioning, 122–23
liberalism, 50, 60, 116–17, 119. *See also* voluntarism, liberal
Lindesmith, Alfred R., 10, 26–27, 30, 34, 82, 133, 159n5; as advocate for decriminalization, 69, 151, 152; critical history of his theory of addiction, 64–71; on desire, 67–68; on dichotomy between mental and physical perception, 4, 27, 63–75, 149–54; on experience, 63–64, 67, 68, 70, 150, 152–53; Galliher-Weinberg debate on, 149–54

poverty, 17, 29, 89, 160n8

practice, 6, 7, 30, 42, 46, 61, 83, 93, 114, 137, 153, 158n2; addiction in, 3, 4, 12, 33, 36, 91, 104, 107, 141, 144; description in, 96; as emergent, 15; Bourdieu and, 5, 73, 126–28; emotions in, 8; intrinsic accountability of, 16, 44, 121; Mol on, 143–44; movements into and out of self-control in, 7; post-humanism and, 11, 35, 139, 140, 147; recovery in, 3, 4, 12; theory and, 12–14, 20, 147; therapeutic, 14, 80, 95

practices of addiction, 136–37, 145

practices of freedom, 4, 123–25, 128, 163n6

praxis, 13, 31, 64, 73–74, 75, 151, 152, 153, 158n2

presentism, 18

principle of charity, 4, 110, 111–12, 113

psychopathy, 118, 119, 132

psychosomatic subjectivity, 5

punishment, viii, 3, 12, 40, 41, 44, 47, 54, 56, 61, 70, 71, 116, 118, 119, 137; Baxter on, 54

Puritanism, 39, 40, 51–55, 56, 59, 157n5

race, 17, 20, 43, 138, 140, 152

Raikhel, Eugene, 42, 46

rational choice, 8, 46, 68, 101, 133, 139; plants and, 48; theory, 8, 32–33, 94, 121, 135

rationality, viii, 8, 13, 29, 35, 46–48, 56, 60–61, 82–83, 95, 99, 100, 102, 117, 136; and emotion, 2, 7–9, 105–6, 107, 114; ideal, 109–13; and self-control, 98, 103–5, 108–9; and social contexts, 112–13

Ray, Marsh, 30, 82, 104, 136, 156n4

reason, 4, 6–7, 14, 132; and freedom, 56, 113, 114; as God given, 55; as historically conditioned, 13, 33; minimum required, 108–9

recovery, viii, 11, 18, 19, 81, 115, 122; ecology of, 81, 90, 159n4; and generalization, 6, 12, 44; as "getting clean," 86–87; particularity of, 12, 43–44, 103–4, 147; in practice, 3, 4, 12; programs, 14, 78, 88, 90, 112–13, 114, 161n2; Benjamin Rush and, 58–59; as self-governed, 85–86, 102; social variables and, 17, 45, 74–75, 118–19, 146–47. See also Alcoholics Anonymous

Reinarman, Craig, 30, 33, 34, 36, 45, 47, 53, 75, 89, 107, 118, 129, 135, 137, 146

Reith, Gerda, 34, 53, 57, 116, 123

relapse, 81, 89, 112, 133; Lindesmith on, 27, 69; Ray on, 136, 156n4; Robins on, 74

reward, viii, 8, 12, 28, 32, 50, 54, 56, 94, 119, 121, 126, 133, 142; and brain circuitry, 45, 47; natural, 9, 11, 44–45, 48, 49, 59, 61; unnatural, 45, 47, 49, 59

Robins, Lee N., 27, 45, 73, 74, 118, 141, 146

Robinson, Terry E., 45, 46, 102, 133

Room, Robin, 17, 31, 33, 42, 54, 75, 77, 93, 107, 131, 135; on normative ambivalence, 28–29, 104

Rorty, Richard, 73, 111, 114; mirror of nature, 13, 138

Rose, Nikolas, 123–24

Rosenbaum, Marsha, 30, 88, 89

Rudy, David, 33

Rush, Benjamin, 77, 116; Christianity and health, 157n4; civic republican, 58; as a father of addiction medicine, 58

Savulescu, Julian, 47, 48, 49

Schmidt, Laura A., 56

Schneider, Joseph W., 33, 69, 77

Schonberg, Jeffrey, 17, 42–43

Schull, Natasha D., 42

Segal, Gabriel, 39, 48, 49, 121; on akrasia, 98–100

self-control, 33, 62, 113, 117, 125, 131, 135, 141, 162n2; addiction science and, viii, 11, 123, 129; ecology of recovery and, 81–82, 90; as emotional restraint, 22, 46, 98, 105–9, 114, 162n2, 163n3; experience of, viii, 12, 86, 89, 105, 133–34, 147; freedom as, 44, 45, 46–47, 114, 162n2; movements into and out of, 2, 3–4, 7, 10, 120; neurology and, 120, 133–34, 147, 162n2; and social context, 109–13; social science and, 135–39, 147; rational coherence of, 98, 103–5, 108–9, 111

slavery, 40, 49, 124–25; addiction as, 54, 55, 56, 57, 58, 60, 61, 62, 92, 116, 128, 137, 139, 142, 147, 157n5

social adaptation, 28, 29, 42–43

social constructionism, 26, 33–36, 78, 83, 135; posthumanism as a form of, 147

social contexts, 8, 13, 18, 33, 56, 61, 84, 105, 116–17, 123, 126, 127, 145–46, 153, 157n5, 158n3; of addiction, 3, 40, 43; of addiction science, viii, 2, 4, 7, 19, 39, 65, 135; akrasia and, 98, 19–113; brain disease and, 119–21; of drug use, 29, 74, 107, 115–16, 118–19, 120, 141, 158n2; rationality and, 112–13; self-control and, 109–13; therapeutic in contrast to scientific, 91, 160–61n10; Wittgensteinian forms of life as, 19, 104. *See also* ecology of addiction; marginalism, social
social science, viii, 2, 9–10, 17, 20, 31, 33, 35, 47–48, 82, 91–92, 95, 116, 129, 135–39, 146, 147
sociology, 25–37, 48, 50, 62, 63, 64–65, 66–67, 75, 91; of science, viii, 2, 18
Stephens, Richard C., 26, 48, 63, 72, 82, 94, 136
subject (human), 9, 11, 14, 16, 35, 36, 62, 128, 135, 140–41, 142, 157n6; fragmented, 62, 125, 126; liberal, 123, 124, 125, 128, 139, 142, 164n6; unified, 62, 125
subjectivism, humanist, 10, 14–16, 31
subjectivity, 10, 14-15, 17, 26, 31, 36, 67, 82, 96; of addicts, 82, 96; Lindesmith on, 67, 153; psychosomatic, 5. *See also* objectivity
suffering, 3, 34, 36, 112, 135, 146, 155n2
symbolic interactionism, 7, 8, 10, 31, 65, 136, 150, 151
Szasz, Thomas, 47, 49, 50

Taylor, Charles, 73, 104
therapeutic community, 77–96, 128
therapeutic practice, 14, 80, 95
therapy, viii, 41, 71, 79, 81, 87, 88, 100, 116, 119, 122, 152
treatment for addiction, 7, 42, 45, 77–96, 98, 100, 112–13, 120, 131, 152, 159n3, 159n4, 159n5, 160n6, 160n7, 160–61n10; as empowering or oppressive, 147; Lindesmith on, 69, 70
Trotter, Thomas, 116; as a father of addiction medicine, 58
Turner, Ralph H., 46
Turner, Stephen, 16
twelve steps, 128, 161n2. *See also* Alcoholics Anonymous

universal, 8, 13, 14, 15, 19, 31, 103, 106, 112, 126; addiction science as, 6, 39–62, 114, 132, 134, 141, 142, 147, 156n1, 162n2, 163n3; Bourdieu on, 19; liberal theory as, 117; particular and, 11–12; rationality as, 109, 110, 111
urban, 58, 145, 160n8

value neutrality, 6–7, 39–62, 156n1
values, 33, 35, 100, 104, 106, 112, 122, 127, 136, 138; in addiction science, 39–62; first and second order, 104; hedonic and eudaemonic, 61, 157n7
Valverde, Mariana, 33, 34, 46, 47, 54, 123, 124, 129, 135
Volkow, Nora D., 39, 45, 129, 133
voluntarism: Blumer's, 69–70, 153; and drug use as choice, viii, 3, 21, 32, 33, 39, 47–51, 53, 137, 159n3, 160n6, 163n1; liberal, 36, 39, 40, 41, 42, 44, 47–51, 56, 59, 60, 61, 123, 124; Lindesmith's, 27, 68, 136. See also *hedonic values*
Vrecko, Scott, 47, 133

Wacquant, Loic, 74, 89; on divided habitus, 127
Waldorf, Dan, 30, 34, 45, 73, 74, 75, 107, 118, 137, 146
Warner, Jessica, 51, 52–53, 55
Waterston, Alisse, 17, 42
weakness of will. *See* akrasia
West, Robert, 32, 129
Whetstone, Sarah, 42, 43
Winick, Charles, 45, 118
withdrawal, 27, 131–32, 133, 138, 141, 156n3; Lindesmith on, 26–27, 67, 135–36
Withington, Phil, 56
Wittgenstein, Ludwig, 1, 29, 73, 114; on family resemblances, 103, 144; on forms of life, 19, 104

Zigon, Jarrett, 42, 46, 61, 156n1
Zinberg, Norman, 72, 118, 141

Chapter 1: "Sociological Perspectives on Addiction." *Sociology Compass* 5, no. 4 (2011): 298–310.

Chapter 2: "Freedom and Addiction in Four Discursive Registers: A Comparative Historical Study of Values in Addiction Science." *History of the Human Sciences* 34, nos. 3–4 (2021): 25–48.

Chapter 3: "Lindesmith on Addiction: A Critical History of a Classic Theory." *Sociological Theory* 15, no. 2 (1997): 150–61.

Chapter 4: "'Out There': The Ecology of Addiction in Drug Abuse Treatment Discourse." *Social Problems* 47, no. 4 (2000): 606–21.

Chapter 5: "Three Problems with the Addiction as Akrasia Thesis That Ethnography Can Solve." In *Against Better Judgment*, edited by Nick E. Evans and Patrick McKearney, 50–69. Oxford: Berghahn Books, 2023.

Chapter 6: "Toward an Ecological Understanding of Addiction." In *Evaluating the Brain Disease Model of Addiction*, edited by Nick Heather, Matt Field, Antony Moss, and Sally Satel, 373–83. London: Routledge, 2022.

Chapter 7: "Post-humanism, Addiction and the Loss of Self-Control: Reflections on the Missing Core in Addiction Science." *International Journal of Drug Policy* 24, no. 3 (2013): 173–81.

Appendix: John F. Galliher, "Comment on Weinberg's 'Lindesmith on Addiction'"; and Darin Weinberg, "Praxis and Addiction: A Reply to Galliher." *Sociological Theory* 15, no. 2 (1997): 150–61.

www.ingramcontent.com/pod-product-compliance
Lightning Source LLC
Chambersburg PA
CBHW030839270326
41928CB00007B/1126